EXERCISE à la Carte

AN ACTIVITY MENU TO A HEALTHIER LIFESTYLE

ASSEMBLE YOUR OWN
ACTIVITY AND EXERCISE
BANQUET
FROM THIS MENU
OF NATURAL TASTY
AND DIGESTIBLE
HEALTHY CHOICES

GEORGE L. DIXON, JR., M.D.

i

Exercise à la Carte: © 1994 by George L. Dixon, Jr. M.D.

Publisher's Cataloging in Publication
            (Prepared by Quality Books Inc.)

Dixon, George L.
        Exercise à la carte : an activity menu to a
        healthier lifestyle/ George L. Dixon, Jr.
        p. cm.
        Includes bibliographical references and index.
        Preassigned LCCN: 94-077596
        ISBN 0-9642615-0-2

        1. Health behavior. 2. Exercise. 3. Physical fitness.
        4. Nutrition. I. Title

RA773.95.D59 1994   613
                                        QBI94-1734

Cover Design: Jerry Wiant Designs, Eugene, OR.
Copy Editor: Jane Kepp, Santa Fe, NM.
Printed in the United States of America by:
                Guynes Printing Company of New Mexico, Inc.
                2709 Girard N.E.
                Albuquerque, NM 87107-1838

Published by: LANE & FORD, Inc.
                1020 Green Valley Rd.
                Albuquerque, NM 87107
                505 344-8755 (Ans and Fax)

Available from: CVT Productions, Inc.
                440 Charnelton,#220
                Eugene, OR 97401
                800 624-4952

DEDICATION

To Margery,
who didn't retire,
for being patient with me,
who did,
over the past five years.

About the Author:

George L. Dixon, Jr., M.D. is an orthopaedic surgeon who retired from active surgical practice in 1989. He remains a Clinical Professor of Orthopaedic Surgery at the University of New Mexico School of Medicine's Department of Orthopaedic Surgery and Rehabilitation. He continues as Consultant for Special Projects at St. Joseph Rehabilitation Hospital and Out Patient Center in Albuquerque, New Mexico.

He is now in his fourth year as medical editor of *Home Fitness Journal*, published by CVT Productions, Inc., of Eugene, OR. He continues to work closely with Mark and Martha Dixon Lange, owners of CVT Productions, Inc., as they continue to guide this video production company through new formats and growth.

He is proud to be a member of the New Mexico Governor's Council on Health, Physical Fitness, and Sports.

Thanks to ever so many.

Jennifer Dixon Hamilton, Registered Physical Therapist, for being gentle, and forthright. **Mark Stodder**, editor of <u>five</u> weekly newspapers, for the smooth compliments before the rougher needed critical aid. **Frances Henslee**, teacher of English, who, I am sure, wonders how I made it through medical school, <u>at all.</u>

Mark and Martha Dixon Lange, who have shared their considerable talents with me through many years. **Sally Dixon Wiener**, my sister, an author and playwright, was finally allowed to review the manuscript with some awe and trembling on my part, because she writes so very well. **Margery Myers Dixon**, my partner and source of loving strength, calm, and inspiration for more than forty years.. **Frank Wesley Dixon**, from whom I have learned much about sales and selling through the years. **Amy Dixon Vargas** whom I dearly love has reviewed it and approves. **Chris McGrew, M.D.**, UNM Department of Orthopaedics, and chair of the Greater Albuquerque Medical Association's Sports Medicine Committee, for reviewing it early on. **Janet Weed,** my greatest fan, took time and energy from her busy life. **Robert A. Robergs, Ph.D.**, University of New Mexico Wellness Center, helped me to accuracy. **Mary Lou Coors**, Administrator of St. Joseph Rehabilitation Hospital and Out Patient Center allowed introduction, time, and tools for my Word Processing learning.

Thanks to **Jerry Wiant** for his remarkable drawings which add clarity to my words.

Special thanks to **Jane Kepp**, my copy editor, for her astonishing ability to get into my skin and brain and make the words come out so well.

To **George Andresen**, President of Guynes Printing Company of New Mexico, a friend and a past patient for his enthusiastic reception of this project.

Exercise à la Carte
Menu Selection

Special Diets: Controlling Your Appetite For Activity

Visit Our Kitchen: Activity Tools In All Shapes & Sizes

Try Us, You'll Like Us: Flavorful Motivators

On The Sofa, Later: Mind, Body And Spirit

Gathering <u>YOUR</u> à la Carte Menu: Customizing Your Plan

INTRODUCTION

In a recent survey by the National Sporting Goods Association, 50 percent of Americans said they were interested in being more active and yet had been unsuccessful in either starting or continuing <u>any</u> increased activity program! Another 25 percent were totally uninterested in any activity, and 25 percent were already engaged in some kind of activity or aerobic exercise.

I wrote this book to appeal to <u>us,</u> that 50 percent of the folks in America who know we need to be more active and eat less fat, but who just can't get it together. I am one of you. Or, I <u>was</u> one of you. Activity and exercise **"à la carte"** has brought new vitality, energy, and interests to my life.

Physical inactivity is four times more likely than high blood pressure or increased cholesterol and three times more likely than cigarette smoking to cause coronary artery disease!

Physical activity of any amount brings HUGE benefits!

In 1993, new guidelines were announced by the Centers for Disease Control and Prevention, the American College of Sports Medicine, and the President's Council on Physical Fitness and Sports:

"Every American adult should accumulate 30 minutes or more
of moderate-intensity physical activity
over the course of most days of the week."

The new message is that activity is <u>normal</u> and doesn't "wear your parts out." It enhances their longevity and the way they function. All your organs and parts work better and longer when you use them but don't abuse or neglect them with too much or too little demand. When you pursue normal, intermittent activities a little longer and more vigorously--for 30 or 45 minutes each day--you have a **fourfold** better chance of avoiding heart and other diseases!

The JOY of having this power and control over the quality of your
life will bring new vitality to your every action.

ix

HOW THIS BOOK CAN HELP YOU GET AND STAY ACTIVE

Our grandparents would react with open-mouthed wonder at even a discussion of our "need" for activity. Their own lives were absolutely filled with needed physical activity: chopping wood, hauling things, cooking, doing laundry with primitive machinery, harvesting, planting--the list is endless.

Along the way to our present sedentary state came fabulous machinery that cooks, washes, changes channels, toasts, opens our garage doors, and all those other things our society loves to do easily. We even have disposable diapers (bless them!). We use our cars to go just a couple of blocks. We do everything in our amazing technological power to defeat our body in its basic cry for motion!

Once you become aware of your many opportunities for bodily motion throughout the day, you can make small, frequent changes in your activities. You need to become more "wasteful" of your fuel and fat stores rather than continue your civilized "energy conserving" behavior. Do all your normal things a little longer and a little faster. As your muscles are called upon to do more work, they will get larger and stronger and use up fuels at a greater rate.

If you can arrange extra activity, exercise, or chores to increase your "activity calories" by 200 over the course of your day, you will benefit by losing fat and gaining muscle.

Everyone at our house loves to eat, so for this book I put activity and exercise into a "menu." I considered small bits of exercise to be **appetizers** and larger activities to be **snacks.** Lunch- or supper-size chunks I call **circuit sandwiches,** and more formal programs--dinner-size activities--are exercise **entrées.** I included **take-out munchies, condiments, indigestion remedies, kitchen gadgets,** and **special dietary needs** on the menu as well.

If you want to lose weight faster, then decrease "food calories" while you increase "activity calories."

But don't think much about the numbers you will find in this book. Just use them a few times to get a feel for the size of the things we will talk about.

With these chapters you can assemble and reassemble your ordinary and favorite sports, work, household chores, or exercises, shaping an ever-changing ACTIVITY MENU that is specially yours and chosen "à la carte."

TO BEGIN:
From Wisdom To Willingness

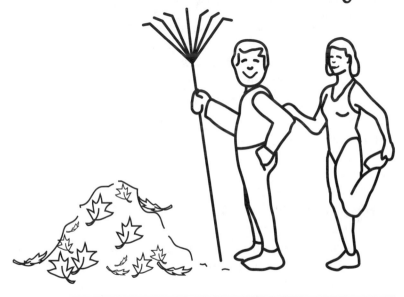

Chapter 1
Appreciating Physical Activity Benefits

WHY BE ACTIVE?

* If you are physically active regularly you will live longer than if you are not. You cannot be immortal, but you can strive to be strong and full of vitality.

* If you are physically active, you are <u>four</u> times less likely to develop coronary heart disease than people who are physically inactive.

* If you are regularly active you will be less likely to get colon cancer, a stroke, or a back injury.
* Regular activity will enhance the quality of your life as you get older and can help you maintain your independence.
* If our schoolchildren are active regularly they will enjoy better health and grades. We need physical education in schools!
* Regular activity will help you control hypertension, anxiety, depression, and high cholesterol, and it may help you avoid diabetes, osteoporosis, arthritis, and diseased arteries.

**Any amount of time you spend being active
is far better than none.
Your benefits increase directly
with the time you spend in activity,
and they increase even faster
as you begin!**

PLEASE SEE "PAR-Q" (Physical Activity Readiness Test), Appendix G.

THERE ARE BENEFITS!

There are **health** benefits and **fitness** benefits from a physically active lifestyle. Both benefits are important. You are invited to become gradually more and more active and collect the huge health benefits that can come to you through simple, moderate activity. Then you may be further lured into regular aerobic fitness activities that promise even more. But get healthy first, then go for fitness.

The **health** benefits of your activity, such as losing weight, living longer, and lowering your risk of heart attack or of fractures due to osteoporosis, are dependent on cumulative, modest, daily activity. You may spread 5- to 10-minute activities throughout the day. You need to be active a total of 30 to 40 minutes to spend an extra 200 calories.

The **fitness** benefits to you, such as increased muscle mass, strength, and aerobic endurance, require higher intensity exercise. The "gold standard" remains 20 to 30 minutes of exercise, 3 to 5 days per week, at 60 to 70 percent of your maximum heart rate. Your effort should be controlled by your target heart rate (see Chapter 9 and Appendix M).

SOME SPECIFIC BENEFITS FROM ACTIVITY AND EXERCISE

Sleeping Better

Staying active during the day invites your body to the natural rest that all animals require. For better sleeping, exercise aerobically two hours <u>before</u> bedtime, because it is too stimulating to let you sleep immediately afterward. There are certain exceptions. Use your bed for sleeping or making love. Read or watch TV from a couch or chair. A quiet time before bed is very helpful (just as you told your kids, remember?).

If you wake up and toss a bit, get up out of bed and sit and read or listen to soft music. If your dozens of problems keep whirling in your head, write them down in order of importance. You will probably find that they become fewer, maybe even smaller. Milk contains calcium and tryptophan, natural substances that cause sleepiness.

Are you getting enough sleep? One of the most serious problems in America is chronic "sleep debt": you have it when you are <u>half asleep all night</u> and <u>half awake all day.</u> Most humans need seven to eight hours of sleep each night. Most experts say to avoid naps. One of the relaxation techniques outlined in Chapter 15 could be very restful during the day. The best way to get more sleep is to go to bed earlier.

There is a natural "high" in humans that begins about eleven o'clock at night and lasts about two hours. So go to bed before this "high," or welcome it and use it.

<u>An increase in your daytime activity is the thing most likely to lead to better sleeping.</u>

Control of Anxiety and Depression

Anxiety and depression can be really distressing, either singly or when they strike together--as they so often do. Activity or exercise is wonderfully effective in helping relieve both. Physical activity is one of the greatest "homeostatic" mechanisms available to your system. That means that it tends to draw your body and mind toward normal.

A rather pure form of depression known as SAD (Seasonal Affective Disorder) comes on in winter, when the sunshine is least, for quite unknown reasons (perhaps it is related to hibernation). Exercise has a good effect on SAD, as does exposure to bright light (daylight bulbs) for about 30 minutes each day (see NOSAD, Appendix F).

The anxiety that accompanies stress (Chapter 15) can often be handled well by a combination of exercise and relaxation.

Anxiety and depression can be remarkably lessened through regular exercise, especially with a friend. A health club setting may offer just the help you need to get started or remotivated.

If your anxiety and depression don't seem to be improved by exercise, please see your doctor. You may need additional help for a while through counseling. There are also presently available very effective antidepression medicines, which are useful even when taken for only a short time. After all, you would wear an elastic bandage on a sprained ankle for a short time, wouldn't you?

Better Sex

Many reports attest to the benefits of activity and exercise in heightening sexual interest and performance. It seems that only men cheating on their wives are likely to die during intercourse! Sex is one of the greatest stress reducing activities known, for both men and women. It can be anxiety producing in terms of performance.

The sex organs are filled and/or moistened by enthusiastic blood flow; exercise and activity can help fill those arteries as well as the ones to your heart, muscles, and brain. Most sexual activity lasts about eight minutes and is remarkably energy demanding!

Intense exercise can make men and women lose interest in sex. In fact, women can exercise so much that their menstrual cycle stops and estrogen levels drop, even to the point at which bone loss (osteoporosis) can occur.

Naturally, the enhanced physical appearance of any vital, active adult is a stimulus to sexual attraction.

Improved Digestion

Contrary to what you may think, moderate exercising will decrease your desire to eat. Activity will help your digestion and particularly help you avoid constipation. Do NOT do hard aerobic exercise within an hour or so after eating, because your blood is directed to your intestines while you digest and may not respond to your heart and muscle needs promptly. But a gentle walk after a meal has much to recommend it--the motion can help your stomach digest food better. You need <u>water</u> and <u>fiber.</u> It is said that eight glasses of water per day are best, but I got pretty waterlogged when I drank that much. Perhaps if you are very active you could tolerate that much water.

Certainly 4 to 6 ounces of water <u>before</u> exercising and 4 to 6 ounces at 15- to 20-minute intervals <u>while</u> exercising are needed. Do not wait until you are thirsty.

There are two kinds of fiber, soluble and insoluble. Many foods contain both--beans, bran, fruits, whole grains, and vegetables, for example. In your intestinal tract, the soluble fiber is thickened and partly dissolved, and some of it used as food--that is, as calories. The insoluble fiber goes through the intestinal tract gathering water for bulk and helping the stool stay soft and easier to eliminate. You need 20 to 30 grams of fiber per day (see Appendix J).

Your **activity** and **exercise** encourage digestion and the passage of material through your intestines. Cancer of the colon (the large bowel) is less likely if your bowel action is faster and more regular. It <u>is</u> possible for you to eat too much insoluble fiber and <u>increase</u> elimination problems.

Beauty = Vitality

Beauty and strength are real partners in life. The graceful, sure movements of people who are filled with vitality are beautiful to behold.

It is not our aging but our "deconditioning," with progressive weakness due to inactivity, that changes our physical appearance. Inactivity and a sedentary lifestyle are the pickpockets of our image.

On the other hand, even if we do manage to get back to our 22-year-old weight and measurements, we will still look older--no major miracles there. But with regular strength and resistance activities, we can reshape ourselves to a remarkable degree. No, not to worry--women won't <u>ever</u> look like World Wrestling Federation members, with bulging muscles!

If you have slowly stopped doing active things because you are weaker, the problem has become a vicious circle. **The less active you are, the weaker you become.** It really is possible to reverse this process at ANY TIME in your life and notice a difference within two or three weeks!

Living Longer and Better

You can alter your time on earth by what you do or don't do while you are here. Reports from both Harvard University and the Institute for Aerobics Research in Dallas show the powerful effects of your lifestyle choices.

Not only your life's length but, more importantly, its <u>quality</u> can be affected directly and successfully by a higher level of physical activity. You can not only postpone your life's genetic end but also keep your vitality more intact closer to that end.

Physical activity is truly an amazing investment!
The more active you are, the better your longer life will be!

WHEN TO BE ACTIVE?

When during the day? Early morning is probably the best time for most of us--except for you folks with allergies, since pollen counts are highest in the morning. Early evening is best for those of you who wish to get away from the tensions of the day, although air pollution is at its height then in most urban environments. Exercise just before bedtime can be too stimulating and may keep you awake. It is best to exercise <u>between or before meals,</u> and doing so will actually decrease your appetite. Right after a heavy meal, exercise may be dangerous to your heart because your blood is diverted away to aid your digestion.

When during life? At any age, activity can only help you--unless you are careless about your limitations. We humans were built physically to <u>move.</u> All your systems and organs work better with daily use.

When during illness? You must use common sense. If you have an illness such as a common cold, or if the weather is bad, choose an indoor activity. Do half as much as you would usually do, or less. Moderate activity enhances your immune system, so it is prudent to continue some of your regular activity habits. Be careful on behalf of your body. If you have <u>special needs,</u> see Chapter 10.

WHERE TO BE ACTIVE?

Outdoor activity is the most stimulating and interesting for us, and is the way our ancestors earned their livelihoods. Sunshine on your hands and face for 20 minutes causes your body to manufacture vitamin D, building better bones. Save the sunscreen until after this brief exposure. The variables of neighborhood, weather, and convenience may lead you to alternate outdoor with indoor exercise.

The increasing danger of our streets needs to be considered in your plans. Often the mugger and the athlete are out at the same time and the same place. Go with others, don't use headphones, be alert, carry identification, and take coins for phone calls. Stay away from brush, doorways, and solitude. Sorry about that.

Indoor activity, either at home or at a health club, gives you control over the environmental variables. If there is instruction at the club, you can control some safety variables. Club exercise can add motivation through group and social contacts.

Home exercise adds great convenience and independence to your program. Activities at home, of course, include that multitude of things we call work or chores.

Now you can consider the same work and chores OPPORTUNITIES for healthful activity!

Studies have clearly shown that if you are active in almost ANY setting you can reach your goals of **health** and **fitness.**

WHICH OF YOUR PARTS NEED ACTIVITY?

There are at least five parts of your human frame that require activity:

* **Your heart and lungs.** The excellent working of your cardiorespiratory system is essential to bring oxygen and nutrients to your brain, muscles, and organs and to remove waste products. Exercise that benefits this system is called "aerobic," or oxygen using, activity.

* **Your muscles.** Muscles need strengthening so that your daily life activities will be easier and safer. Strength, endurance, and neuromuscular grace, coordination, and balance are needed to prevent injuries. Aging muscles respond very well to demand, if coaxed. Strong muscles use more fuel, which includes fat.

* **Your joints.** Along with muscles, joints need stretching and full use in the greatest range of motion possible. More flexible muscles and joints, together with stronger muscles, make you quicker and less likely to be injured in daily demands. Graceful, controlled, strong

motions are a sign of your <u>vitality.</u>

* **Your brain.** Brains are subject to the "use it or lose it" rule. Studies show that you can improve creativity, memory recall, retention, and speed of new learning with physical and mental activity. When you are more active, your brain gets a better blood supply and can respond faster and better to the large and small challenges of life.

* **Your social self.** Social interaction is necessary to us all. As your physical parts are used, your ability to reach out to others to help, to learn, to change, or to accept will increase. You will not be "too tired." Activity <u>begets</u> activity.

HOW TO BE ACTIVE?

This book will help you by offering many activity and exercise choices from which YOU choose what YOU LIKE. Assembling your own "**exercise à la carte menus**" can be fun!

The calorie numbers are **unimportant.**
The time you spend being active is **more important.**
What is **most important**
is that you **become** and **stay** active!

Step into Chapter 2 and start to fill your activity plate!

LIGHTER FARE:
A Little Activity Goes A Long Way

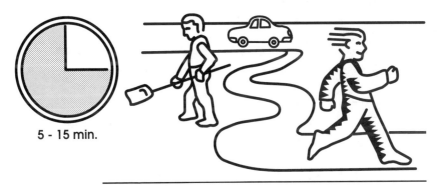

5 - 15 min.

Chapter 2
Appetizer Motions

A little appetizer motion, taking just two to four minutes, will help you get your parts in gear and soon be ready for more. It can be just a taste of a later **bigger bite.** Please, "graze" throughout the day, repeating these motions as you wish. Try to fit these kind of bites in as part of your normal flow of activity. Look around you, and you will find natural bites of action everywhere.

 * Take a set of ten steps, up and down, one second per step.

 * Walk briskly for three minutes.

 * Get up and down from a chair five times; use your arms and the chair's only if you need to, or if you want to add strength to your arms.

 * Whenever you sit, sit down and stand up two or three times.

 * Stretch your arms all the way overhead five times.

 * Take as many "unnecessary" steps as possible during your day.

9

Carry a smaller load that will require two or three walking trips instead of one. **Radical?** Yes--quite different from our usual efficient ways of doing things economically. Use a few seconds more and reap a bushel of benefits!

* Take five DEEP breaths, way in through the nose and way out through your mouth. Relax after each one for three seconds.

* Hang the laundry outside on the line.

* Get a good cordless phone and walk around while talking. Talk as long as you can walk!

* Get off and on elevators a floor or two above or below your level and climb up or down.

* Park a block or two from your work or errand and walk.

* Keep weights of two to five pounds in your auto. Use them two to four minutes twice a day.

* Take two- to five-pound weights to work with you and keep them in your desk. At least twice a day use them for three minutes. (A one-liter plastic bottle full of water or soft drink weighs about two pounds.)

* When you accompany a friend to the mall, walk around rather than sit while your friend does personal shopping.

* Don't slouch. Mom told you to stand up straight! It is not instinctive; it is learned. Let your head move up on your lengthened neck and tuck your chin in a little. Your body will align itself. Smile!

* Gluteal muscle (buttock) exercises will help keep your posture correct. Put your chest up and your chin back. Squeeze your buns together as often as you think about it! You can do it standing in grocery lines or bank lines, at a stop light, even sitting or lying down. It can be done in any position! And no one knows you are doing it.

* Tighten your buttocks and stretch your legs before you get out of bed in the morning--it gets your body prepared for weight bearing.

You can think of lots of ways to use appetizer motions throughout your day! Move with the kids or with your dog. Walk some apples over to the neighbor's house. Do "commercial motions" while watching TV. The KEY is to do more activity in small, easily chewed doses. Try a little nibble every hour while you are getting used to the idea. Soon you'll be ready for some delightful **ACTION SNACKS!**

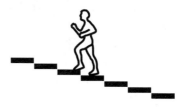

LIGHTER FARE

Chapter 3
Action Snacks/A Bigger Bite

These "action snacks" take from 5 to 15 minutes. If you use ONLY action snacks, you can pick the ones you like and plan to use up those 200 extra "activity calories"* per day. Mix and match--do different ones every day! Sure, you can do multiples! Scatter them throughout your day. You can snack at home, at work, or at play-- **"exercise à la carte"**!

* 15 minutes of window washing (50 calories)
* 10-minute stationary bike trip (75 calories)
* 10 repetitions of bent-knee abdominal half sit-ups, called curls (60 calories)
* 15 minutes digging in the front yard (90 calories)
* 8 minutes of jumping rope (90 calories)
* 10-minute walk at lunch. Go one-half mile, or six blocks--three blocks out, three blocks back. Go with a friend. (60 calories)
* l5 minutes of raking (50 calories)
* 15 minutes of push mowing (50 calories)
* 10 minutes on a treadmill (60 calories)
* 15 minutes of mopping (50 calories)
* 15 minutes of softball (40 calories)
* 15 minutes of chopping wood (90 calories)
* 15 minutes of tennis (singles--70 calories)
* 15 minutes of vacuuming (50 calories)

* 15 minutes of sweeping to upbeat music (80 calories)
* 10 minutes on that mini-trampoline (90 calories)
* 10 minutes of dancing (you remember how!) (80 calories)
* 15 minutes of hanging clothes (40 calories)
* 5 times up and down 10 steps; 4- to 6-inch steps; single step or real stairs (90 calories)
* 15 minutes of golf (40 calories)
* 15 minutes of making beds (40 calories)
* 5 minutes on a stepper machine (80 calories)
* 15 minutes of sexual activity (50 - 90 calories)
* 15 minutes spent ironing (35 calories)
* 15 minutes of shopping (50 calories)
* 10 minutes at pick and shovel work (100 calories)
* 15 minutes of inline, roller, or ice skating (80 calories)
* 15 minutes of steady swimming (60 calories)
* 15 minutes of running (150 calories)

For a brief discussion and help with some of these topics, if needed, see Chapter 4, Circuit Sandwiches.

---

* Dr. Robert A. Robergs tells me these are more correctly called "kilocalories." But I will leave them "calories" since that term is more familiar.

Be A "TRY ATHLETE"

TRY WALKING for your legs and heart.

Start with five minutes, three times a week. Add 2 minutes per week for 6 weeks, then add 2-3 minutes per week for 6 more weeks.

GOAL: 2 miles three times a week at 12 weeks.

TRY STRENGTHENING your arm muscles.

Start with 2 pounds of weight in each hand (a pint of water=one pound). Bring hands up to face level bending elbows - 5 times at once, three times a week for 2 weeks. Then 10 times. Then more weight.

GOAL: 10 pounds, 10 times, three repetitions, three times each week.

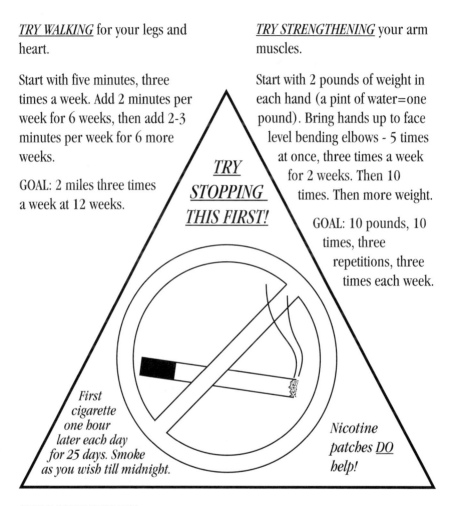

TRY STOPPING THIS FIRST!

First cigarette one hour later each day for 25 days. Smoke as you wish till midnight.

Nicotine patches DO help!

TRY EATING LESS FAT.

Start with 2% milk for a month (whole 3% milk for babies up to 5 years - their brain needs it). Then mix 2% with 1% for a month (Go slowly for family cooperation). Then 1% for a month. Then skim ½% or less milk.

GOAL: Less than ½% forever!

MORE FILLING:
Activity Selections For The Heartier Appetite

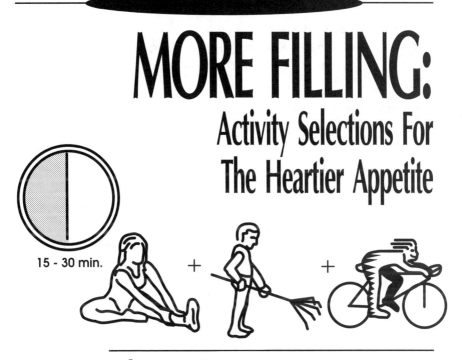

15 - 30 min.

Chapter 4
Circuit Sandwiches/Freshly Made

These activity "sandwiches" are made with a variety of ingredients that are reasonably well balanced. You may vary them by picking any four segments you like, or doubling any one and taking away another, or putting them in any order--or you may do them just the way they are. Combining them this way, you will be doing a "circuit"-- think of it as if you were walking around a buffet table and building a sandwich from your four favorite ingredients. Your goal can be to collect 200 "activity calories" or more each day. Sure, they can be mixed with the **"Action Snacks"** in Chapter 3!

The calorie estimates are for approximate body weights: 155 pounds for men and 130 pounds for women. The less weight you have to carry, the fewer calories you burn per unit of time. The difference is hardly important. The principle is to move your body frequently!

Each ingredient takes five minutes. Together they make a 20-minute sandwich that burns 85 to 115 calories. See Chapter 12 for more information about exercise machines and equipment.

* **Walking**
  Abdominal Curls
  Stretching
  Stationary Bicycle   **(100 calories)**

WALKING (30 calories). Use good court shoes or shoes by SAS, Rockport, or another quality manufacturer. Start with five minutes daily if you are not used to walking. Outside is grand but walking around the house or the mall is just fine.

When you get used to the mall or outdoors, add two minutes each week for six weeks. Then add two to three minutes each week for another six weeks, and by about the twelfth week you will be walking 1.5 to 2 miles in 30 minutes! If you listen to music while you walk, 3.5 miles per hour (MPH) will correspond to about 120 beats of music per minute (BPM).

The calories you use up are based primarily on the distance you move your body (that is, your weight) and secondarily on the speed with which you move it. Move your body faster to use more calories per unit of time. A slow jog or a fast walk of 4.5 to 5 MPH will use 100 calories per mile. You can use up those same 100 calories by walking slower and longer.

Race walking is more than simply walking faster. It involves easily learned but exquisite techiques. Your feet follow a straight line in front of you. One foot is always on the ground. It is low impact. Lots of hip and spine motion is required. Contact your local walking club or your library to learn about the race-walking folks.

Jogging is slow running. As you become used to walking faster, at about 4 MPH or a little more you will probably start thinking of breaking into a run. Do it! Count 50 running steps and then walk again until you want to jog again, usually for 50 to 100 steps. Repeat as you wish, "à la carte." TWO CAUTIONS: First, if you have anatomically abnormal legs or back, be very gentle and slow at switching to running steps. Second, pay attention to your "rate of perceived exertion," or RPE (see Chapter 9). As you add more and more jogging and running time, you will prefer more flexible running shoes.

Try a couple of one-mile community group walks or jogs. I'll bet you will do fine and be proud.

Running is cleansing and exhilarating and necessary and lots of other great things. Do seek information from a local group, a friend, or the American Running and Fitness Association (Appendix F).

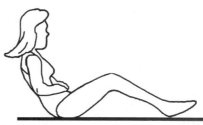

ABDOMINAL CURLS (15 calories). These used to be called sit-ups. Put your arms across your chest, <u>not</u> behind your neck. Bend your knees. Do one quarter sit-up. Hold it for a count of three. Exhale while doing it. Let yourself slowly down. Wait for a count of three, then repeat. Start gradually, with three sit-ups, and increase to ten. DON'T say, "I'll start with 20 and work up." That is a sure recipe for failure!

STRETCHING (15 calories). Walk around for about two minutes to get your blood flowing to your muscles. Stretch any muscle enough to feel tension, not pain. Hold it for 10 to 15 seconds, push it a little more, then hold 10 to 15 seconds more. Breathe easily. No bouncing. Then relax. Start with your arms overhead, then put them behind your back. Stand and bring either foot toward your buttock, stretching your front thigh muscle. Stand leaning into a wall with one foot forward, the other foot back, and stretch the back calf by lowering its heel to floor, GENTLY. Stop when you feel that pulling behind and just below your knee. Stretch just once or twice, several times daily.

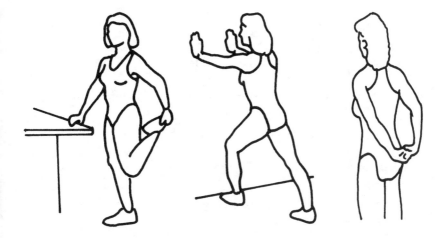

STATIONARY BICYCLE (40 calories). Your down leg should be slightly bent at the knee. Sit straight. Go for more revolutions, less tension at the beginning. Cycle for five to ten minutes, once or twice daily.

* **Stationary Bicycle**
  Stretching
  Free Weights
  Abdominal Curls   **(90 calories)**

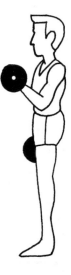

FREE WEIGHTS (20 calories). Beginning strength training is called <u>isotonics</u> (see Chapter 12). Start with two-pound weights and do eight repetitions of each exercise, then repeat the whole thing, so you do a total of two "sets." If it feels easy, increase the repetitions to twelve; then increase the weight at weekly intervals. Do free-weight exercises every other day.

Plastic gallon milk or water jugs, full, weigh eight pounds. Take some out if that is too much. Stand or sit with the your arms hanging down, holding the weights, and bring the weights up slowly (2 - 3 seconds) until you are bending (flexing) your elbows. Take longer (4 - 5 seconds) to straighten (extend) your elbows. Do this five times, rest, and do it five times more if you are not feeling the strain. Do this exercise every other day. Next week, slowly add more weight and more repetitions.

* **Walking**
  Deep Breathing
  Stationary Bicycle
  Stretching   **(100 calories)**

DEEP BREATHING (15 calories). Take a deep, full breath in through your nose, then exhale it slowly out through your mouth. Wait three seconds between breaths. If you get dizzy, STOP!

* **Abdominal Curls**
  Walking
  Push-ups
  Stretching   **(85 calories)**

PUSH-UPS (40 calories). Get on your hands and knees, bend your arms, and lower your body down as far as you can and still push yourself back up. Start with as many as you can do--ONE, if that's all. If this is too easy, balance on your hands and <u>toes</u> and bring your body down and up with your arms alone.

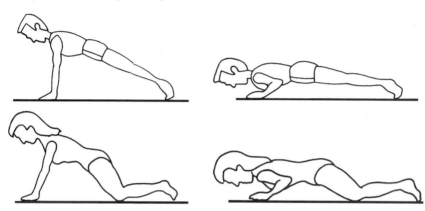

* **Stretching**
  Stair Climber or Bench Step
  Abdominal Curls
  Free Weights   **(95 calories)**

STAIR CLIMBER (45 calories). These machines are hard work! Stay flat footed. Great for your buttocks and calves. Take one step per second. See below for bench stepping.

* **Walking**
  In and Out of a Chair
  Stationary Bicycle
  Stretching   **(115 calories)**

IN AND OUT OF A CHAIR (30 calories). Find a chair with a straight back, a firm seat, and arms--not a deep, soft chair. You need to have enough room to bend your knees to get your feet back behind the front edge of the chair. If you find it too hard to get up using your legs alone, start by using both your arms and the chair's, then progress to getting up and down <u>gracefully</u> using just your legs. Start with sitting down and getting up five to ten times. Don't PLOP back down into the chair!

* **Stationary Bicycle**
  Stretch Bands
  Walking
  Deep Breathing   (105 calories)

STRETCH BANDS (20 calories). These oversize rubber bands usually come in three strengths. Start by reading the directions! They are wonderfully portable. Sometimes bands are included with a video.

* **Stretching**
  Rowing Machine
  Stationary Bicycle
  Free Weights   (105 calories)

ROWING MACHINE (40 calories). Hard work! Start carefully. Using a rowing machine may harm your back if it is already sore.

* **Indoor Skiing Machine**
  Stretching
  In and Out of a Chair
  Abdominal Curls   (105 calories)

INDOOR SKIING MACHINE (40 calories). Lots of coordination is needed to use these machines--it will take you five to seven days to master the technique. Poles are easier. Indoor skiing machines offer the lowest impact and high returns. Follow the directions!

* **Abdominal Curls**
  Jump Rope
  Deep Breathing
  Free Weights   (100 calories)

JUMP ROPE (50 calories). Your rope should be long enough to reach under both feet and up to your armpits. Hold the rope with your palms up, elbows close to the waist. Start with an easy pace and jump or jog at a two-count beat. Start by jumping for 30 seconds, walking for 30 seconds, then jumping again. Jump on a mat or thick rug. Five minutes is a hard job at first. This is the highest impact ingredient!

* **Bench Stepping**
Slideboard
Stretching
Walking   **(150 calories)**

BENCH STEPPING (40 calories). This is a very inexpensive way to get the exercise of a stepper or stair climber machine. Bench stepping is very aerobic, with medium to low impact. Beginners: use a four-inch platform, look down every few seconds, plant your heel firmly on the bench, don't bend your knee more than 90 degrees, and don't pivot on your bent knee. Fine video help is usually available when you buy the bench.

SLIDEBOARD (60 calories). These inexpensive boards are growing in popularity. Basically a slideboard is a smooth, slick sheet of tough plastic, three to four feet wide, with blocks at either end. You stand on it, wearing socks but not shoes, and slide sideways until the block stops you. It's a little like indoor ice skating. It offers very low impact but requires about twice the energy of walking. This activity goes great with music, videos, or TV. There are no reports of injury yet, but squatting is liable to make your back, knees, and heel-cord hurt sometimes. Start carefully.

ATTENTION:

Before eating any of these sandwiches, walk around for one or two minutes, take a couple of deep breaths, and stretch your joints a little to get the blood flowing to your muscles.

Some of these sandwiches can be done with enough speed and vigor so that by moving quickly from one to the next--around your circuit--you can achieve an aerobic effect, keeping your heart rate in your target heart rate zone. Please see the discussions of heart rate in Chapter 9 and Appendix M.

Look over and consider the mellow suggestions in Chapter 15 as counterpoints to these "circuit sandwiches"!

MORE FILLING

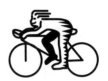

Chapter 5
Main Course/Entrée

By now you have enjoyed **appetizers** and perhaps an **action snack** or a **circuit sandwich,** and are ready for the **main course!** You can be proud of yourself for having become active and aware that adding a main course to your "exercise à la carte" menu is not only possible but of great benefit!

The ideal main course improves both health and fitness by providing heart and lung conditioning and by strengthening--enlarging--your muscle fibers. Those fibers will then consume fat calories more effectively.

You need invest only 30 minutes, three days a week, in activities that raise your heart rate to between 50 and 85 percent of your maximum heart rate, and then 30 minutes two days a week strengthening your muscles with weights and abdominal curls. This modest investment will provide a lifelong bounty of **HEALTH** and **VITALITY!**

(Your maximum heart rate equals 220 minus your age. See Chapter 9 for a discussion of heart rates. Also see Appendix M for more discussion of target heart rate zones, and Appendix G for PAR-Q.)

MENU CHOICES

(See Chapter 12 for a detailed discussion of equipment)

DON'T BE LAZY, SUSAN (220 calories)
Spend 30 minutes, including stretching for 5 minutes and then **stationary cycling,** which includes warm-up, cycling for at least 12 minutes at target heart rate, and cool-down.

KEEP STIRRING (250 calories)
Spend 30 minutes, including a brief warm-up, brief stretching, then **walking** for 25 minutes or **stair climbing** for 15 minutes, followed by cool-down walking.

SNOW CONES (250 calories)
Spend 30 minutes, including a brief warm-up and stretching, 20 minutes of **indoor cross-country skiing,** and finally a cool-down.

OUT THE WINDOW (250 CALORIES)
Spend 30 minutes to **walk** a mile and a half or more. Your target heart rate should be 60 percent or more of maximum heart rate. A treadmill will work just fine. Use a slight "up" incline.

THE STEW POT (100 - 150 calories)
Spend 30 minutes, including a brief warm-up and stretching, then arm muscle exercises using free or fixed weights; abdominal curls; and leg exercises with gravity, ankle weights, or fixed weights. Finish by cooling down with a brief walk. (NOTE: This is not aerobic exercise but is wonderful for building muscle fibers and strength.)
A "circuit" of these exercises can be done briskly and can usually keep your heart rate up in the aerobic range.

A PARTY! (200 calories)
Spend 30 minutes at ballroom, cowboy, or line dancing or rock aerobic low-impact dancing. Videos are fun. More fun is line dancing. Most fun is dancing with a partner.

SMOOTH AND FROTHY (200 - 250 calories)
Spend 30 minutes at freestyle swimming, AQUAJOGGER water walking or running, or aerobics in water. (A fine book on calisthenics comes with the AQUAJOGGER; see Appendix E.)
Water provides l2 times the resistance of air in all directions. Water is also very supportive and is great for after injuries, bad backs and

neural dysfunctions. When walking, start in shallow water that comes to your upper thighs or waist. Deeper water is much harder. Walk backward and forward a few steps. Stay on your feet, not just on tiptoes. Don't lean forward. Swing your arms.

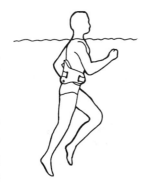

For a really hard workout, try treading water using only your legs! Stay vertical, keep your hands at your sides or on your head, and, with your kicking, rise up out of the water. Careful: 30-second blasts, with 30 seconds in between, for 8 or 9 minutes will be plenty.

KEEP THE COOK WARM (250 - 300 calories)

Spend 30 minutes chopping wood, shoveling snow or wet earth, hand mowing, or running up and down stairs repeatedly. Be careful with that first snowfall, it's heavy. Moving it could provoke a heart attack, so take your time!

SPORTING EVENTS

Racquetball, squash, handball
30 minutes = 300 calories.
Good for agility, endurance, reflexes. Quite aerobic for brief intervals.

Tennis, singles
30 minutes = 200 calories.
Same as above. Doubles are less.

Downhill skiing
Long runs, bumpy: 30 minutes = 300 calories.
For legs and arms; great for endurance, balance.

Roller skating, rollerblading, or ice skating
30 minutes = 300 calories.
Great for legs and aerobic exercise.

Badminton
30 minutes = 200 calories.
For agility, reflexes; arms get good use.

Golf

30 minutes = 100 - 150 calories.

You burn more calories if walking, still more if wheeling your bag, and even more if carrying your bag.

Rowing

Outdoors: 30 minutes = 400 calories.
Indoors: 30 minutes = 350+ calories.
Overall trunk, arms, and legs get a terrific workout.

Nordic skiing

Outdoors 30 minutes = 400 calories.
Indoors 30 minutes = 350 calories.
Hardest workout. Low impact. Lots of sweat.

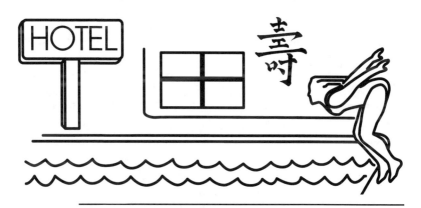

TAKE OUT & EXOTIC:
Activities To Go-From Near And Far

Chapter 6
Take-Out Munchies/On The Road Again

You are not home all the time. When you are not, you still have to be somewhere! This is a collection of nibbles to take with you in your travels.

IN YOUR CAR

* Stop your car at least every hour, get out, walk around for two to five minutes, do three half-squats and five overhead stretches, and then get going again.

* There is an audiotape you can follow for exercises in your car when you are stuck in traffic or when you are <u>not</u> driving. Call for the "Collage Video" catalogue--phone number in Appendix C.

* Keep two-pound weights in your car to use during traffic jams or when you are stopped for whatever reason.

IN YOUR HOTEL

* Elastic band sets come in varying strengths, often with directions,

and they are light and pack well.

* One-liter (or one-quart) plastic water or soft drink bottles weigh about two pounds when full of water (a pint is a pound), but they can be filled to your desire to serve as free weights. A one-gallon plastic milk or water jug, when full, weighs eight pounds.

* Most hotels have steps for you to walk up and down. Most will offer advice on nearby walking or jogging paths, sometimes with maps. Go with someone if you can! Avoid headphones on unfamiliar routes. Be alert.

* A jump rope fits easily into a briefcase. It should be long enough to go from armpit to armpit around both feet. Jump for 30 seconds; then step in place for 60 seconds; repeat three times or more as you are able.

* Use the hotel pool. If you don't swim or don't want to get your hair wet, stay in the shallow end and walk back and forth. Ask at the pool desk for an AQUAJOGGER you may rent or use.

ON THE AIRPLANE

* When you are on airline trips, drink six to eight ounces of water hourly--the air on a plane is very dry. Get up every 30 minutes or so, stretch to the ceiling, and walk back and forth to the lavatory even if you don't need to use it. (You probably will if you drink that water.) Avoid overuse of alcohol. This is essential on long, overseas flights to avoid foot and leg swelling and possible vein inflammation.

* Save your reading for the flight, and take a walk between connections. Yes, sometimes that does become a run.

* Reach up toward the ceiling every 20 to 30 minutes. Push against it. Reach behind your head and stretch your elbows back.

* Think your way up from your toes and tighten your muscle groups one at a time as you go, on one or both sides of your body. Working your way up, squeeze your abdominal muscles, your buttocks, your shoulders, and so on, up to your neck. This is called isometric exercise: your muscles tighten but your joints don't move much.

TRAVELING IN GENERAL

* You always take your abdomen with you anyway, so do some abdominal curls (sit-ups) with those muscles. Lie on your back with your knees bent and cross your arms over your chest. Curl your body about one-quarter up toward your knees. Exhale going up and breathe while holding the position for about five seconds. Relax back down for another full inhale and exhale, and then repeat 5 to 20 times.

* Unless you walk up or down on them, bypass all escalators in favor of stairs. Be careful though--it is dangerous and probably illegal to go opposite the flow on escalators.

* For a good lower back and buttock stretch, stand an arm's distance from a sturdy chair back or a low countertop. Hold on. Keep your feet flat. Keep your back straight and lean forward a little. Bend your knees, pushing forward through your hips, pressing your buttocks together behind you until you are in a half squat. Squeeze your buttocks tightly and don't let your back arch as you come up to standing again. Try for five times.

* Stretching is grand. Walk a little (two minutes) to get your blood flowing. Then gently stretch any group of muscles. Don't bounce. Hold the stretch for ten seconds, then stretch a little more and hold it for ten seconds. I like to start by stretching my arms overhead. Then I stretch my calves by leaning forward with my hands placed on a wall; I put one leg back and put that rear heel down, slowly, to feel the pull in back of and just below my knee. Careful, you can overdo it and make your calf sore. Relax and then do the same on your opposite side. Do this calf stretch twice, no more.

* When you exercise on the road, be easy on yourself. Stick to the same kinds of things you do at home if you can, and do only about half as much.

* The behind-the-back pull is wonderful for your upper back, neck, and shoulders. Sit or stand straight, head on long neck, with your shoulders low. Stretch your right arm overhead and back down your neck and spine. Bring the other arm around and up from below. If they meet, hold them clasped for 20 seconds and then change arms. If they don't meet, put a sock or handkerchief in your right (upper) hand and grasp it with the left (lower) hand. Stretch one arm gently with the other, then change arms. Do several sets.

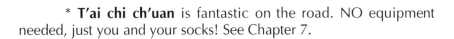

* **T'ai chi ch'uan** is fantastic on the road. NO equipment needed, just you and your socks! See Chapter 7.

TAKE OUT & EXOTIC:
Chapter 7
A Far East Flavor

No menu would be complete without these wonderful and exotic offerings. They will bring new interest to your activity efforts.

Many of the "soft" exercises, as opposed to "hard" ones, have a Far Eastern flavor and an ancient, almost prehistoric essence. At least, we think of them that way, even if historical fact would prove differently.

T'AI CHI CH'UAN. Twenty-five hundred years ago this martial art was developed by people who watched and duplicated the graceful, efficient, and sometimes deadly movements of animals. The lessons of quiet, inner strength are taught by movements named "Snake Creeps Down," "Repulse the Monkey," "Part the Wild Horse's Mane," and similar things. T'ai chi is very low impact and completely portable, and you can learn it from a book or, better, from a video. The best way is the ancient way, by a master's example.

YOGA. The origins of yoga are lost in time, but the main framework dates to the second century B.C. The "Eight Stages" are to be supervised by a guru. Yoga refers to a number of different ways to salvation.

The main physical stages are three and four. The variant schools developed in medieval India are those of Spells, Force, and Dissolution.

For every pose, there is an opposite pose. Complete balance of movement, stretching, and deep breathing are emphasized in these exercises, which tone up both Mind and Body.

Every yoga class is different. There is no national accreditation. You need to know that there are flowing types, dance types, very strenuous aerobic blends, and those that are quiet and meditative. There are books and several videos (see Appendix C) concerning all stages and schools of yoga, and the best way may be for you to read about it a bit first and then get into it.

PILATES METHOD. If you have posture and movement problems, here comes the reformer. With the Pilates Method, you <u>will</u> move correctly. Stretching and strengthening muscles is important. Visit a teacher or your library.

ALEXANDER TECHNIQUE. A method that will teach you how to align your body and move efficiently while being mindful of motions and correcting them.

BALLET, MODERN DANCE, AND FREE-FORM MOVEMENT CLASSES. All of these can help you shift to <u>full circles</u> of motion from the <u>linear</u> motions done in most "hard" exercise routines.

FAMILY DINING:
Relationships: Fat, Fuel, Food & Fitness

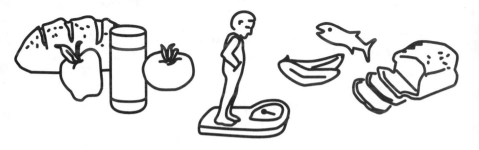

Chapter 8
The Perfect Couple/A Jack Sprat Family

I'm too heavy for me to lift! The problem is that you have been nibbling at activity a little but mostly you have been <u>thinking</u> about doing something about it. You have never really bitten into an activity menu with a commitment to continue.

Of course you will have to eat less if you are overweight, but not a lot less--mostly, just less fat! What you have to do is to use more of your fuel regularly. You are very economical in your body activity, a trait that probably came to you genetically. You will have to learn to be more active!

Activity and exercise will not simply make you hungry--actually, quite the reverse happens, for reasons not well understood.

How fat are you? Pinch that extra tissue at the side of your abdo-

men, the back of your thigh midway from hip to knee, or the back of
your upper arm. Sit slumped forward, look down at that roll, and
grasp it with thumb up and fingers down to gauge the thickness. Each
roll should be one inch thick or less. Each quarter inch beyond one
inch means about ten pounds of extra fat.

How much should you weigh? A Stanford Medical School study
suggests that women should multiply their height in inches by 3.5 and
subtract 108. Men should multiply their height in inches by 4, then
subtract 128. (To me this seems about 10 to 20 pounds light for people
over 50.)

Why do we have these fat glubs all over our bodies? It is to store
energy; they are your pantry. You know that fat contains about twice
the calories (9) of carbohydrate or protein. It does so in those glubs
inside your skin too. Nature arranged those portable and wonderfully
economical stores against the variations in food available to our ancestors, so they wouldn't run out of fuel when times got hard. We
continue to store fat nowadays, even though we eat regularly. If we
had to store that amount of fuel in watery solution, we would weigh
300 pounds!

The 1990 dietary guidelines from the U.S. Department of Agriculture assess waist-to-hip ratios. Your waist should be smaller than your
hips. Excess abdominal fat is more dangerous to your heart than buttock and thigh fat. Pear shape is safer than apple shape.

You cannot trick your body into selectively using up its fat stores
either generally or locally. **The only way to lose fat is to burn more
calories than you take in.** Muscles do use their local fat stores for
energy.

Research continues into local fatty area reduction, but no techniques have been successful so far. Recent reports of thigh reduction
with applied creams are most likely wishful thinking.

Dr. Dean Ornish tells the most up-to-date truth in his book Eat
More, Weigh Less. He says it's what you eat, not how or when, that
makes you fat and prone to heart and blood vessel problems. He is
part of a rapidly growing school of belief that fat is the main villain in
our diets. His book points out how you can beat this killer. I recommend it highly.

Jeffrey Fisher, M.D., a cardiologist from New York, reports in the
magazine Bottom Line Personal that "a man needs 12 calories per

pound of body weight to sustain his daily needs (a 180 pound man needs 2,160 calories) and a woman needs 11 calories per pound." You can lose weight by eating less, and eating less fat is the most effective way to accomplish that.

In general, the more liquid the dietary fat, the less polysaturated it is, and the better it is for you. Plant oil is better than animal oil. But the most important thing to understand is that you must limit all fats! The slickest way into weight loss--dietary fat reduction--is also the quickest way to healthy eating.

SOMETHING TO THINK ABOUT

There are about 550 grams in one pound of human fat.

There are 9 calories per gram of fat.

There are 3500 calories per pound of pure fat (plus water).

If you increase your activity by 200 "activity calories" per day, using the suggestions in this book, it will take **18 days** to lose that pound of fat.

If you take in 200 "food calories" fewer in fuel per day, using the simple suggestions in this book, it will take **18 days** to lose that pound of fat.

If you do **BOTH**, you will lose that same fat pound in just **9 days!**

If you change your life just this little bit each day, you will lose **40 pounds** of pure fat in one year, while you replace lots of that weight with fat-burning muscle!

AT THE UPPER END OF THE SYSTEM

Meanwhile, at the "fuel intake" end of the system--your mouth--you must replace fat with complex carbohydrates (pasta, breads, rice, and cereals) and high fiber foods. You need soluble fiber, which can help lower blood cholesterol, and insoluble fiber, or roughage, which helps you avoid constipation and colon disorders (see Chapter 1 and Appendixes H and J). Under stress, men tend to eat less and women more, especially sweet and bland foods.

Start lowering the 40 percent or more of fat in your diet down to 20 or 25 percent slowly, as you get used to things tasting differently. Covert Bailey has wonderfully simple suggestions such as low-fat salad dressing, mustard, or nonfat yogurt on that baked potato. Spread mayonnaise on your bread and then scrape it off, leaving the taste without the volume. Use alternatives and substitutes: applesauce for oil in baking; olive oil for butter; egg whites (or egg-beaters) for whole eggs; nonfat yogurt for sour cream; air-popped popcorn for potato chips.

Dr. Ornish says lower it all at once to 10 percent, and you will lose the craving and the sense of missing the fat in your diet in a few short weeks. Tough order! But any effort to approach a 10-percent fat level in your eating can only help you. He says that you can eat often and until you are full, if you don't eat fats and do eat mostly vegetables. He states that the closer you get to a fully vegetarian diet, the healthier you will be. Read the first 80 pages of his book--it might save your life!

Skim milk is awful if you are used to whole milk, which is more than 3 percent fat. Go to 2-percent milk for a month. Then mix 1-percent and 2-percent to get 1½-percent milk for a month. Then go to 1-percent and even to ½-percent, and then, if you wish, move on to skim milk. If the whole family is involved slowly, success is more likely.

Chew sugarless gum while you cook--it helps you sample less. Stop saying "diet" food and refer to it as "healthy" food.

Eating smaller meals but eating more often is felt to be one of the secrets of keeping intake under control. In fact, there is evidence that snacking steadily on the right things (mostly vegetables) will keep you from eating everything in sight. A steady supply of energy is best.

One way of eating more slowly is to put down your fork or spoon between each bite, to use up time. It takes 12 minutes for nourishment to reach your brain centers to tell you when you have had enough. Fast food, eaten fast, can get far ahead of that message and your needs. Try doing all your eating in one location, or eating as much as you wish but only one helping.

Replace red meat with white meats. Cook chicken with the skin on, then take it off. The meat stays moist; the fat stays with the skin. Cook hamburger meat, then pour off the grease, gently squeeze the meat in a paper towel, rinse it for a few seconds in water, and then reheat. Much of the fat will be gone!

Try replacing some of the hamburger meat with mashed beans or cooked grains. I just tried a recommended concoction of two parts ricotta cheese, one part peanut butter (no hamburger), and it was okay, at least with strawberry jam!

The new labels on food products make it much easier to figure the calories per serving and then to figure the percentage of fat in that serving (see Appendix N).

You can figure your daily food intake for a few days to get an idea of what percentage of your whole diet comes from fat. Most cookbooks have charts indicating the nutritive value of foods. Count all food calories and divide by the fat calories, and you will know roughly how much fat you need to cut out of your diet in order to come close to the 30 percent fat intake that many experts consider to be healthy.

STARVATION

Zero is not better!

Those fat stores have been accumulating to take care of you if you are threatened by starvation, and your body is much too clever to use them up first. Instead, muscles shrink away first because your body "eats" them up. They require too much energy to operate if you aren't getting enough food. A pound of muscle requires about 40 calories a day to stay alive! Fat is much less expensive--it needs only 2 calories per pound per day for survival. (That's one reason you are trying to increase your muscle mass--to use up calories!) Your body also decreases its basal metabolic rate against a long fast. So fat is used last and slowly, which is why starvation is a poor way to diet.

When you do start to eat again, your body stores away as much fat as possible. Amazingly, going just 18 hours on empty, by not eating breakfast, stimulates your body to start storing fat!

There is comfort in the research reports that a bit of stoutness is far preferable to going constantly up and down 15 to 20 pounds in what is called "yo-yo" dieting--which is downright dangerous to your heart's health. More fatty stores are encouraged with each episode of starvation and replenishment.

If you are seriously obese, PLEASE see your doctor before you begin any program, even these simple suggestions!

THE EXERCISE PLATE

Slower but longer

You need to commit to exercising <u>longer</u> in order to encourage your body to use its fat as fuel. The best exercise is aerobic, at a lower target heart rate (45 to 60 percent of maximum heart rate; see Chapter 9), but for a much longer time. During your first 15 to 20 minutes of activity, your body uses glucose for fuel; then it switches to fat. Instead of 20 minutes of aerobic exercise, three times each week, you will need 40 to 60 minutes, four to five times per week. Just walking along fairly briskly for that much time is perfectly fine.

Your body uses up muscle first when you diet, because fat costs your body less to maintain. If you make your muscles work and demand food, your body will then turn to your fat stores for the fuel. As your muscle fibers strengthen and increase in size, your metabolic rate will increase and your fat stores will be used up more rapidly. **Even when you are not exercising, more muscle uses more fuel!**

Certainly, you can burn more calories faster by jogging, running, or bicycling faster. But because you need to exercise longer, the faster rate will likely increase your injury rate too. That's a bummer--then you can't even do things slowly! So, long and slow is the way to go. Remember, start gently!

One villain is our sedentary lifestyle. As we get older, we are less active, and our muscles shrink while our fuel intake stays the same or even increases. Slowly our bodies take on a higher percentage of fat. The good news is that the situation is always reversible. Muscle fibers do not turn into fat; they are right there waiting for us to become active once again!

Decrease the fat in your diet.
Increase the activity in your life.

Simple diet and simple activity are the PERFECT couple!

SPECIAL DIETS
Controlling Your Appetite For Activity

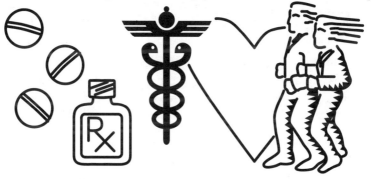

Chapter 9
Exercise Disorders/Avoiding Indigestion

Overexercising, pigging out, must do, too fast, too soon, too big a bite, too often, too little--you can get "exercise indigestion" that may even cause you to drop your valiant efforts to lead an active life. It is important to learn how to prevent painful symptoms at home, at work, or during sports.

Too soon? Estimate your safety factors before starting any activity plan. See Appendix G for PAR-Q, a simple test that will help you judge your physical activity readiness.
* Don't be bullied into any exercise plan.

Too fast? Don't attack the activity menu as if you were trying out for the Olympics tomorrow.

* Start slowly and gently. (Take small bites.)
* Invest slowly if you want expensive equipment (see Chapter 12).

Too much? "If a little is good, a whole lot must be better." Not true!
* "No pain, no gain" went out a decade ago. It was and is a harmful
concept and practice. Muscles and joints can be injured.
* "If I can't exercise, I'm a bear to live with." Too much exercise can
become a kind of addiction. "Obligatory" exercisers need to vary their
routines and times in order to break the addiction. Their chance for injury
is high, and the compulsion to "push through" and go on to further damage is extreme.

Too often? Using the same favorite exercise every day has the same
effect as always eating the same thing. Some muscles and joints are
neglected, and some are overworked. Vary your exercise. Sets of muscles
need rest. Cross-training is the by-word.

Pigging out? "This is so easy, I'll have a couple more helpings!" Muscle
repair and construction takes from 48 to 72 hours, and it can't be
rushed.

SUN TANNING

Indoors or out, sun tanning presents special hazards. There are two
types of ultraviolet light, UVA and UVB. They have different charac-
teristics, but both damage you. It was once thought that UVA, the
light most commonly used in tanning salons, was less harmful, but
researchers have discovered that it, too, can cause long-term and cumulative damage leading to skin cancers. Tanning salons in general
are not well regulated, nor are their machines well calibrated. Even if
they were, the damage still occurs.

It is best to use a **sunscreen** with SPF (sun protective factor) of 15 or
more and a combination of ingredients that protects you against both
UVA and UVB rays. Wear a hat, especially from ten o'clock until two
o'clock.

WATER

As an ordinary-size, inactive adult, you should drink about two
quarts of water each day (12 8-ounce glasses). There is abundant water
in juices, fruit, milk, and most foods, so you probably get at least half
of that water in your diet. Don't count beverages with caffine or alco-

hol, because both are diuretics--for every glass you drink, you urinate out about a glass and a quarter. If you are on medication, especially "water pills," please check with your doctor because this may be too much water for you.

The best way is to drink water regularly throughout the day. You will need to drink 6 to 8 ounces 15 minutes before exercising and, depending on the temperature, 4 to 6 ounces every 15 minutes. You sweat a lot while exercising, even in winter. Indoor exercise also requires fluid replacement at the same regular intervals. Do not count on your human thirst indicator, which is not well developed, to warn you. By the time you are thirsty, it is late in your need for water.

Unless you are working very hard, very long (1½ hours or more), and/or it is very hot, you do not need "sports drinks." But those drinks do taste better than water to most people, and water does get absorbed faster when it comes in 6-percent glucose solutions. Salt tablets are rarely needed except in extreme heat conditions.

AVOIDING OVERUSE PAINS

At work, at home, and at sports

"Syndromes" are collections of symptoms that occur together. Some common ones: cumulative trauma syndrome, repetitive trauma syndrome, and overuse syndrome. They are not the same but are related. The first two are usually associated with upper extremities and a workplace setting. The last is usually a lower-extremity problem in a sports setting. Both can occur, rarely, even at home. Lower back problems can happen in any setting!

Painful symptoms may be caused by too much bodily motion, either too fast or in an awkward position, without enough rest time between cycles of motion for soft tissue, muscles, tendons, and ligaments to recover their normal elasticity.

Examples of true high-repetitive use might be 20,000 key strokes per hour, 12,000 knife cuts per shift, or elevation of your arm overhead 7,500 times per shift.

Low-repetition jobs have a cycle time of more than 30 sconds, less than 1,000 cycles per shift, and fewer than, say, 2,000 hand manipulations per shift. These jobs rarely cause symptoms.

Most jobs are NOT highly repetitive and carry little risk of this kind of injury. Some jobs do ask for motions that may place joints and muscles at the extremes of their range of motion and can cause symptoms of overuse.

Many symptoms are caused by stresses at home, with family or in other relationships. They can also occur because of stresses at work. You must recognize the part stress plays in your pains and try to decrease it (see Chapter 15).

CARPAL TUNNEL SYNDROME

Carpal tunnel problems have been known for 200 years but have burst into prominence with the "repetitive trauma" concept in worker's injuries. The carpal tunnel is the route many tendons take to get from your arm into your hand. The tunnel has bones on three sides and a thick ligament on the fourth. The tendons are hard, and the median nerve is soft. Any extra pressure in the tunnel affects the nerve first. This pressure can cause numbness of the thumb, index finger, middle finger, and half of your ring finger. Onset may be related to needlework, painting, sewing, writing, typing, racquet sports, power tools, and driving for long periods.

Fracture of the wrist, obesity, pregnancy, some infections, and an underactive thyroid can all contribute to the problem.

There are some things you can do to avoid carpal tunnel syndrome. Roll up a towel and place it under your wrists when you are working at a keyboard, or use one of the commercially available pads. Exercise and stretch your hands during the day at rest periods. Clench, release, and stretch your hand out fully five times. Stretch your wrist and hand back by putting your whole hand on a tabletop and bring your forearm up to about an 80-degree angle to the table top, gently, three to five times.

Save your hands by doing after-work activities that don't stress your hands--walking, jogging, bicycling, indoor skiing, and so forth.

Take breaks every 45 minutes or so and stretch your hands, as well as your wrists, elbows, and shoulders. Stronger muscles and correct posture decrease your chances of having carpal tunnel problems.

Try to separate any job or social dissatisfaction from your physical symptoms.

Wrist splints can be worn at night to keep your wrists from bending too much in your sleep, which puts pressure on the soft median nerve in the carpal tunnel (that is why those fingers go to sleep). Some of my patients wore them for months and even years, only at night, and they had far fewer symptoms in the daytime. Your doctor can suggest careful doses of vitamin B_6. Your carpal canal can be injected with cortisone, which often helps for a long time.

Surgical release of the carpal tunnel is a very common operation in America. Surgery is successful 93 percent of the time, which is very good, unless you are among the 7 percent who don't do well. Just be sure you have tried everything else first.

LOW BACK PAIN

Low back pain is nearly the most common painful human problem, second only to dental cavities!

Don't smoke: it diverts blood away from your discs, those pads between your vertebral bones, and weakens them. Don't slouch. Get up from sitting every 30 to 45 minutes and move your body.

Lift things with your knees. Squat down, embrace the object, hold it close, tighten your belly muscles, and then stand up. You will really be surprised the first time you do this; there is almost no feeling of strain. Stand close to a shelf if you have to lift something onto it. It seems clear that those black corsets with suspenders do help prevent back symptoms, probably because they are a constant reminder to lift correctly! They also indicate that some instruction has been given in proper lifting.

Get rid of the extra weight you have in that "belly pack" in front of you. Strengthen the muscles of your abdomen with abdominal curls. When you work standing, as you do when ironing, standing in an assembly line, or working at a kitchen counter, put one foot up on a low (four- to six-inch) block or stool. That is why the bar rail was invented--so people could stand and drink longer.

Get down on one knee when picking up your grandchild or infant from the floor. Pull your foot up to your lap when you are sitting to put on your shoes and socks--don't bend over to the floor. Avoid lying on your stomach, but if you do, put a pillow under your abdomen and pelvis.

Change your mattress every few years; turn it over every few months. Don't watch TV in bed unless you have huge pillows to prop up your whole back and neck and head. Pivot when you get in and out of an auto by keeping your legs together and trying to take both feet off or put them on the ground together.

John Sarno, M.D., at New York University School of Medicine feels strongly that most of our back, neck, and shoulder pains stem from our inappropriate response to anger. He calls this tension myositis syndrome (TMS). Have a good examination first, to be reassured that nothing is seriously wrong, and then talk yourself out of the pain or get psychological help to do so. Sarno's book is titled Healing Back Pain (see Appendix A).

See your doctor early if you have acute back pain. Keep moving, even if you just do a little walking three or four times a day. A tub is too hard to get in and out of, but hot showers help. Medications really help early on. Ask your doctor to arrange at least two learning sessions with a good physical therapist, one early and one later. You need to learn posture and lifting and be taught exercises for trunk muscles--which you then do until you get to be 107 years old!

New studies show that walking activities and/or low-impact aerobic exercise can reduce your chances of getting low back pain and can assist greatly in rehabilitation after an acute attack is over.

TENDONITIS

Tendonitis is inflammation of a tendon sheath, which can occur when a motion is performed continually and very rapidly, always at the same angle, or at an awkward angle or approach. One way to avoid it is to vary that approach or angle as often as you can, and change tasks as often as you can. Avoid stretched or odd positions at the end of your joint's range of motion.

Tendonitis also can happen where tendons wear out. Such places are the shoulder, elbow, hip, heel-cord, and the bottom of your foot near the heel. All respond pretty well to decreased use, ice, and anti-inflammatory medicines such as Ibuprofen.

NECK AND SHOULDER PAIN

Neck and shoulder pains may come about from stress coupled with a static position held for too long a time. To help avoid pain, get a pad for your telephone so that your neck doesn't get all crooked over for hours. Change ears, or get an ear piece. If you can't get the boss to buy the equipment, get it for yourself--it's your neck!

Stand up for a good stretch and some shoulder shrugging every hour, or even more often. Step around behind your chair and do five half-squats, then go up and down on your toes five times. Do this at least two or three times each day.

Reach overhead with both arms, reaching high so that your biceps touch your ears, about five times, four times a day.

Take two- to five-pound weights to work with you and keep them in your desk. At least twice a day use them for two or three minutes. A one-liter plastic bottle of water or soft drink weighs about two pounds.

Too <u>much</u> neck motion can produce problems too, especially if you are less fit or older. Avoid looking up, especially fast, hard, and all the way up. It may cause you to faint or give you a very sore neck. Replace that motion with a slow, gentle, "not-all-the-way-up" motion.

Just as it causes low back pain, repressed anger is an important and common cause of neck and shoulder pain too.

* Do your best to separate any anger, job dissatisfation, boredom, or home, family, or coworker problems from your physical symptoms. It is hard to separate your body from your brain. Sometimes your brain can convince your body to feel ill. See Chapter 15 for more on stress reduction.

**Say something nice to somebody each morning
and each afternoon.**

Smile!

OTHER OVERUSE PAINS

Overuse injuries are common in sports settings. They are related to the cumulative or repetitive trauma syndromes but are not the same. The difference is that overuse injuries are usually lower-extremity problems in a sports setting, and the repetitive trauma syndromes are usually upper-extremity problems in a worker's compensation setting.

You can bring pain on in several ways during activities: by a direct injury; by overuse of a normal body part; and by normal use of an abnormal body part. You and your doctor can sort these things out.

* **Hip joint** problems or tendonitis in the front or groin can be a tendon or a true joint condition. Pain at the side of the hip is usually a tendon problem, and may be caused by a short leg. Pain in the buttock most often is from the lower spine, not from a hip joint.

* **Knee** problems often stem from muscle imbalance, improper shoes, or anatomical abnormality. They may be be caused by overuse of the same running route, or by squatting too deeply.

* **Shin splints** are usually caused by too much work, done too soon. They often result from using improper shoes for a particular activity.
* **Heel pain** at the cord can be from direct shoe counterpressure. A small 1/8-inch lift inside the shoe is worth a trial. Heel pain under the heel bone often comes from inflammation of the <u>plantar fascia,</u> a tissue band that bowstrings across your arch from toes to heel. Hard floors and improper shoes can cause and aggravate the inflammation. Insoles or orthotic devices can often help.

NONSTEROID ANTI-INFLAMMATORY DRUGS

These over-the-counter medications--called nonsteroid because they do not contain cortisone--include Aspirin, Ibuprofen, the newer Aleve, and similar drugs. They clearly decrease soreness when you take them before or after activity. All of them have a certain number of side effects, even at small doses. Just because they are sold without a prescription does not mean they cannot harm you, even when used in the doses recommended on the package. Read and follow the directions. There is recent evidence that the "expected" amount of muscle strengthening may not occur following this useful pain relief. Perhaps a <u>little bit</u> of pain is needed for gain after all!

CHAIRS

Sit comfortably erect, not slumped forward or backward. Your back support should tilt. The chair seat should be adjustable. You should sit with your feet flat on the floor and knees bent at least 90 degrees, so that they are level with or even slightly above your hips. A small foot rest can be used intermittently for good relief of strains. Use a contoured seat. Your chair should provide support for three-quarters of your thigh. Obtain arm rests if possible. Get out of that chair at least every 30 minutes to move about and stretch.

An **ischial wedge--**a rolled towel just behind your sitting bones but under your buttocks--can provide amazingly good relief of postural back strain. If you alternate the wedge with a **lumbar roll,** you can vary your spinal posture often and relieve strain. If you work at a video display terminal, you may be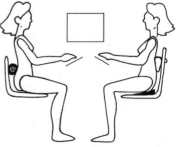

helped by adjustable seats, glare-free screens, and rest breaks. Ergo-nomics training and apparatus, if needed, can help decrease your chances of any body parts becoming painful.

I recently saw a useful computer program for Windows and DOS called "Exercise Break." It provides simple moving graphics and in-structions on how to keep muscles limber while sitting at a work sta-tion (see Appendix E for the address and phone number).

HEART RATES

A Guide to Your Appetite for Activity

You can find your pulse low down on your neck or, even bet-ter, at your wrist near the base of your thumb. Your wrist pulse is easier to find when you are working hard. Pressure on the big artery high in your neck, just below your jaw, can slow your pulse and be a problem.

You may count your pulse beats for l5 seconds and multiply by 4; for 10 seconds and multiply by 6; or for 6 seconds and multiply by 10. All will give you beats per minute. When you start out, count longer--you will be more accurate. Later you will do fine with a 6-second count.

Electronic pulse meters are accurate enough when they count from your finger or ear lobe. If real accuracy is essential, then a chest strap will count your heart muscle contractions electrically and transmit that information to your meter. This kind is much more accurate when you are outdoors working hard.

The normal, healthy human heart beats 72 times per minute. A lower heart rate can result from being a consistent exerciser, from some medications for heart or blood pressure problems, or from the fact that you simply came that way.

Your **resting heart rate** can be measured by recording your pulse before arising on two different days and averaging the figures. If your rate is less than 50 or more than 90, please check with your doctor.

Your **maximum heart rate** is age related. Take 220 and subtract your age. That rate is as fast as your heart should safely be encour-aged to beat.

Your **target heart rate zone** is 50 to 85 percent of your maximum heart rate (see Appendix M). Target heart rate is an estimate of exercise intensity, measured in heartbeats per minute. (There are other ways to measure exercise intensity, but this way is clear, and even I understand it!)

If you are just starting your healthy activity program, aim for 50 to 60 percent of maximum heart rate. If you are a moderate exerciser, try 60 to 70 percent. If you are in great and improving fitness condition, go for it at 70 to 80 percent or more. (See Chapter 16 on goals.)

Your pulse rate should be back to normal within eight to ten minutes after exercising. If not, you are working too hard.

RATE OF PERCEIVED EXERTION (RPE OR BORG SCALE)

As you become more active, you will recognize that sometimes you are really working hard, sometimes not hard at all, and sometimes you are just coasting. This awareness of your exertion level is quite an accurate measure. Pay attention to your own perceptions! You may have a number of other clues such as hard breathing, fast pulse, or profuse sweating, but your overall perception is usually right on. You will be most accurate at the upper and lower edges of the table below.

NOTE: Medications that control your heart rate and response may mislead you. Ask your doctor about this <u>before</u> exercising!

What you perceive (RPE)	What your pulse is doing
0 = resting	
1 = very, very light	
2 = very light	about **50 percent** of maximum heart rate
3 = light	
4 = moderate	about **60 percent** of maximum heart rate
5 = moderate	
6 = somewhat hard	about **70 percent** of maximum heart rate

7 = hard
8 = very hard   about **80 percent** of maximum heart
                                       rate

9 = very, very hard
10 = maximal

Usually a workout between RPE levels 2 and 4 (very light to moderate) is satisfactory for **health** purposes. For ordinary **aerobic fitness**, aim for levels 4 to 7 (moderate to hard). **Athletes** should go for 7 to 10 (hard to maximal).

SPECIAL DIETS:

Chapter 10
Exer-dietary Needs/Special Diets

What you bring to the table is important, especially if you bring special needs and conditions. Your need for increased physical and mental activity is essential, no matter how fragile or complex you feel your life has become.

The joys of being stronger and more in control of your life are possible no matter where or when you start. So start now!

These notes about special needs will help you feel more confident about not making any of your problems worse.

They do not and will not replace the critical advice your doctor or other health care partners can give you.

ARTHRITIS

There are two main kinds of arthritis, osteoarthritis (OA) and rheumatoid arthritis (RA). The former is restricted to joints, usually the hips, knees, and base of the thumb. The latter is an overall disease that affects the joints as well as almost every other tissue and part of the body.

It is clear that excess body weight contributes to the onset of OA, especially in women's knees. For example, even ten pounds of excess body weight increases the forces of going up and down stairs by 60 percent.

While it is important to keep your joints moving, it is essential to lower their impact work by steadily getting rid of extra weight. Your joints take one million steps carrying that weight every year!

If you have OA, start your activity plan slowly and gently, probably in warm water to get a good range of motion. You may also begin by stationary cycling or walking for five to ten minutes every day, working up by adding one or two minutes per day each week, up to about 30 minutes (at about 12 weeks). Your own doctor, or an M.D. called physiatrist, or a physical or occupational therapist can advise you about specific exercises. There are grand new medicines if pain is a real problem. Tylenol has been reported to as effective for OA as almost any prescription medicine.

RA is different. Dealing with it means serious learning of your own fatigue limits and techniques of joint protection. A physical therapist or physiatrist can help greatly. If you have severe RA, start with isometric exercises (just working your muscles against gravity, with minimal joint motion); if your condition is less severe, exercise in a warm (90 degrees or hotter) pool, or try walking or stationary cycling. Avoid high-impact or running activities. T'ai chi ch'uan (see Chapter 7) can be a great help.

Start slowly and listen to your body. If pain increases and persists two hours after exercising, slack off. Be sure you can do easier exercises for a week before moving on. Stretch and move your joints each day.

The Arthritis Foundation, either at the national level or your local chapter, is a real gold mine of information (see Appendix E).

DIABETES

Activity and exercise three days weekly, along with weight control, have been shown to decrease your chance of developing adult-onset (type II) diabetes by more than 20 percent. Regular aerobic exercise does increase muscle mass and will often decrease your insulin dosage. Talk with your doctor <u>before</u> lowering your insulin dosage!

When you start to exercise, check your blood sugar before and after your workout. You will need to begin slowly and have someone with you, so that if you become hypoglycemic, help is right there. Carry glucose with you. Inject your insulin into a quiet place, usually the abdominal wall. Avoid exercise when diabetes control is not good. Avoid exercising when insulin is reaching its peak. A good time to work out seems to be 30 to 60 minutes after you eat, while your blood sugar is high.

Dietary saturated fat is bad for you for three reasons: gaining weight, increasing coronary risk, and increasing insulin resistance. Eat less of it.

As you start your walking program, be especially careful to select well-padded, comfortable shoes that are big enough to allow for thick socks. You may have insensitive feet, and they are much easier to keep free of blisters than they are to heal.

No high-impact exercises are allowed. It is even possible that you are in the small group of people with diabetes for whom even moderate exercise may be too much. For example, you must take special care if you have problems such with the eyes (retinopathy), kidneys (nephropathy), or bones or joints (arthropathy).

YOU MUST CHECK CHANGES IN EXERCISE, DIET, ORAL MEDICATIONS, AND ESPECIALLY INSULIN WITH YOUR DOCTOR!

PREGNANCY

Ordinary activities, modest sports, and low-impact aerobics are good for both mother and child after the fetus is firmly implanted. This is usually after the second missed period if you have had no spotting. Abdominal and back work up to the third trimester can bring comfort. Avoid exercising on your back after the first trimester; it decreases the blood supply to your baby. Also avoid prolonged times of motionless standing.

Walking is probably the best exercise. If you were very inactive before becoming pregnant, be prudent about starting an exercise program. Talk with your doctor. As your abdomen increases in size, your center of gravity will be different and your balance may be affected. Partial weight-bearing exercises such as stationary cycling and cool-water swimming are the safest ways to continue exercising throughout your pregnancy.

Avoid hot tubs or saunas.

The main danger to your baby during the first three months is overheating. If your temperature, taken orally, reaches even 100.4 degrees (38 degrees C), the heat may harm your baby's developing brain and spinal nerves. You **can** reach that core temperature by overexercising! During the the third trimester, more than 15 minutes of moderate exercise competes with your baby for blood.

Don't forget to take multiple vitamins, especially folic acid. It is for your baby's spine and nerves. Ask your medical partner.

During your last two months, do any of your exercises within 30 minutes after eating to avoid drops in blood sugar, which is bad for both of you.

After your baby arrives, breast feed or pump before exercising, because your baby will not like the lactic acid--waste products of exercised muscles--in your milk.

Your postpartum weight will likely drop to within 5 pounds of your normal weight if you haven't gained more than the 25 or 30 pounds your doctor advised. Stretched abdominal muscles will respond to easy and then more enthusiastic abdominal curls.

The American College of Obstetricians and Gynecologists has published an exercise guide (see Appendix F). Your personal exercise history may allow you and your doctor to fashion a considerably more active program.

HIGH BLOOD PRESSURE

Regular activity and exercise will often help to control modest increases in blood pressure and will certainly decrease the dosage of any medicine required to control it. Lifestyle changes are important whether you need drugs or not. Drug therapy continues to evolve to decrease side effects such as impotence. Both systolic and diastolic hypertension need attention.

It is reported that a ten-pound weight loss will often lower your blood pressure by five points.

Unless you have it measured, you will not know if you have high blood pressure until it is too late! It gives NO warning!

Various high blood pressure medications have profound effects on your body's response to exercise. You must talk with your doctor before beginning an exercise program, and with each medication change.

Improper exercising can temporarily elevate your blood pressure--for example, if you strain without breathing out properly (as you are likely to do during abdominal curls), or if you start too fast on any machine, especially steppers. A hard, fast start to an exercise on a very cold day can also elevate your blood pressure dangerously--be careful when shoveling snow.

Riding a recumbent stationary bicycle is reported to be less likely to elevate your blood pressure than riding an upright one.

CORONARY ARTERY DISEASE

This is what you are trying to avoid by being active, doing aerobic exercises, and paying attention to your diet.

There are some conflicting data about antioxidants, but the basic advice about supplements still remains valid: 6 to 15 milligrams of beta carotene; 200 to 800 I.U. of vitamin E; and 250 to 500 milligrams of vitamin C.

Exercising after a heart attack, angioplasty, open heart surgery, or even cardiac transplantation can help you recover and avoid the recurrence of artery disease. Careful medications and dietary measures (LOW FAT, HIGH FIBER) help too. Both strengthening and aerobic exercises can help lift the depression that often follows a brush with mortality. Your program must be guided by your doctor.

A similar shutdown of the blood vessels in your legs--peripheral vascular disease--can often be relieved by persistent, daily slow walking, to tolerance, with brief rest periods. Ask your doctor if this is appropriate for you. Aquatic pool exercises, if the water is not at too high a temperature, can help blood flow into and out of your legs. After a surgical opening of the blood vessels of your legs, walking can help keep the vessels open.

OSTEOPOROSIS

Osteoporotic bone is chemically normal, but it is thinner and weaker because there is less of it. From age 14 to 35, if you exercise or are reasonably active, you are making your bones stronger. From then on, especially during the six years following menopause, your loss of bone is steady and can be dramatic in more than one-third of women. There may be a genetic reason for osteoporosis. Men become osteoporotic too, but they do it at a later age, mainly because they start with heavier bones.

You can prevent much of the accelerated loss surrounding menopause and later in life by taking adequate calcium (1,500 milligrams) and vitamin D (400 units), doing regular weight-bearing exercises (three times a week), and eating a good diet. It is clear that estrogen replacement therapy (HRT) is the best way to prevent rapid bone loss. Other medicines and therapies are available, but none is so well documented as estrogen. It has some dangers along with its bone- and heart-saving virtues. So talk with your doctor about hormone replacement therapy if you are approaching menopause or have had surgical removal of your ovaries.

Exercise must be weight bearing to be of any stimulation to your bones. They are living tissue and respond to demand like the rest of your parts. The astronauts, weightless in space, lost amazing amounts of calcium. Their bones thought they had been retired and melted away. Aquatic exercise, although great for sore joints and gaining muscle and even for an aerobic workout, is not weight bearing. An exercise bike is partly weight bearing. Walking is totally weight bearing.

You can find dietary calcium most easily in dairy products. You will need about 1,500 milligrams of calcium per day, all your adult life. You probably take about 800 in your diet, so a supplement of 500 to 1,000 milligrams is probably good to take. Take the calcium with meals. One glass of milk, skimmed or whole, has about 300 milligrams. If dairy products do not agree with you, try the new calcium-fortified orange juice--it contains 300 milligrams per 8-ounce glass, just the same as milk! Low-fat yogurt contains much more calcium than an equal serving of cottage cheese. It is possible to take too much calcium: more than 2,000 milligrams per day is too much. Too much calcium does not cause arthritis but can calcify arteries and cause kidney stones.

Vitamin D can be provided by 20 minutes of sunshine on your hands and face per day. It causes your body to produce 200 to 300 milligrams of vitamin D. An additional 200 to 400 units of vitamin D should be taken by mouth. You must have it to digest the calcium, and your bones also use it. Vitamin D is toxic in amounts of more than 2,000 units daily.

The most important reason to take good care to have strong bones is to prevent later fractures. Wrist and spine fractures are painful, but the real devastation comes with a fracture of your hip. Mortality from this injury is 10 percent, and the chance of losing your independence is 50 percent!

When you are being active and building or maintaining bone, you are also gaining muscle strength and stamina as well as keeping your good balance and coordination. All these things add up to decreasing your chance of falling and breaking your hip. What a BONUS!

OBESITY

See Chapter 8, The Perfect Couple

ARTIFICIAL JOINT REPLACEMENT

Because your new joint is artificial, it starts wearing out at the moment of "purchase and installation." It cannot repair itself the way your natural body can. You, as its host, are in a race to see which of you outlasts the other. If you are young and use it very hard, you will probably need it relaced again before you die. If you are older and use it wisely, it will likely last as long as you need it.

You have the choice. The same exercises, done more gently, that are good for your natural parts, are good for your artificial joint. There are certain cautions to be observed with each particular joint.

Hips. Avoid bringing your hip up bent (flexed) to more than 90 degrees, a right angle. Stay out of deep chairs because you tend to bend forward much farther than a right angle and then struggle to get up. This puts too much strain on the joint and it may dislocate. Use the pool steps to get out of the swimming pool--the ladder forces you to bend your hip too much. Don't cross your legs at the knees; it is all right to cross them at the ankles. Don't bend over from the hips while keeping your knees straight. Avoid straight leg raising. When doing knee and thigh (quadriceps) strengthening exercises, be sure your thigh remains supported.

Walking and bicycling are both very safe and helpful in getting and keeping muscles around your hip joint strong. Moderation is the keynote. Jogging and running impact the joints with up to four or five times your body weight. Your artificial joint can't take it. Don't do it!

Knees. They respond the same way as hips to impact work--don't subject them to jogging or running or aerobics with impact. Rule of thumb: Keep one foot on the floor at all times to control impact. Don't force the joint's range of motion; do encourage it steadily. One degree of gain each day will give you a useful range in 90 to 100 days.

Elbow and **shoulder** replacements are very good at relieving pain. They are not as good at restoring an almost normal range of motion as are hip and knee replacements. Unless you simply have to, do not use artificial finger, wrist, elbow, or shoulder joints for weight-bearing purposes such as walking with crutches or getting up from chairs.

The same joint-protection techniques used to make your natural, painful joint easier to live with will also extend the life of your artificial joint.

The best exercises following joint replacements are water supported and no impact, with many repetitions and light tension or weights. Realize that your artificial joint can rarely approach your normal joint in functional range. Remember that the pain has been wonderfully relieved! Be gentle and use that new joint often.

LOW BACK PAIN

See Chapter 9, Exercise Disorders

WEATHER EXTREME PROBLEMS

Cold

Winter is a lovely and tough time of the year. It is a time of rest for most plants and animals. It provides an extra set of problems for you, demanding solutions. It is a grand time of year for cross-training, so that you are outdoors enough to savor the season and indoors to do good and safe exercising.

Do not wear clothing as if you were going to sit outside. Wear at least three layers. The layer next to your skin should be of polypropylene or some other "wicking" type of material. The next layer can be a sweater of some kind, and the outside layer should be windproof and have vents available. As you bike or run or walk outbound, do it into the wind so that your return trip, when you are likely to be sweating, will be warmer.

It is said that you can use up more calories when you are active in the cold because your body not only has to provide the energy for your muscles but also has to keep you warm. Start out much more slowly in really cold weather, because a sudden rise in blood pressure can occur.

Lots of body heat is lost through your uncovered hands. Mittens are best. Two pairs of socks in those older shoes that are a bit large will be better than one. Shoes with neoprene collars are dry and warm. The greatest heat loss--up to 40 percent--will occur through your head, so wear a cap big enough to protect your head, neck, and ears. Vaseline on exposed surfaces will help protect them.

Your lungs will not freeze because the air will be sufficiently warmed on its way down. But asthma can be very "cold sensitive," and you may precipitate a bad spell of bronchospasm.

You can get much colder than you realize, especially running or bicycling, because you add speed to the wind chill factor. You can get frostbite of the ears, nose, lips, fingers, penis, or nipples. The holidays are no excuse to quit! Do your walking at the mall. Cut down to less than half of your regular program, but don't stop-- you will need the stress reduction, and you need to spend those extra calories. Don't do heavy exercise just after a big meal. A slow walk is fine; otherwise wait two hours. Take extra vitamin D during the winter--200 units extra daily (for a total of 400 units)--because your rare sun exposure may not produce enough.

There is an odd but real condition known as SAD (Seasonal Affective Disorder) that comes with the shorter and darker days. It causes true depression in some folks. Exercise and exposure to a bank of fairly bright lights (daylight spectrum) for some time each day helps a great deal. Try setting up your exercise machine in front of a light box. (See Appendix E for the address of NOSAD, the National Organization for Seasonal Affective Disorders.)

The greatest modern answer to cold weather exercise is not to "work-out" but to "work**in**"--indoors, that is. Your stationary bicycle, indoor cross-country ski machine, treadmill, or stair climber provides a great workout. If only you could get rid of the boredom. Well, you can, with "point-of-view" videos made to solve just that problem. You can be bicycling in Maui or Vermont; skiing in St. Mortiz or Colorado; or climbing out of the Grand Canyon! See Appendix C for information about "Destination Fitness" workout videos.

Heat

The splendid summer brings quite another set of problems. We know that water is lost all the time from our bodies in sweat and respiration. When the temperature is high, our bodies are cooled by the evaporation of sweat. If the humidity is high also, then our sweat cannot evaporate and we can easily become overheated.

You must drink plenty of water each day: six to eight 8-ounce glasses. Before exercising, drink 6 to 8 ounces, and then 4 to 6 ounces every 15 minutes or so. Do not wait to become thirsty. Your human ability to gauge your thirst is not good, and you can be far behind in water needs. Juices or sports drinks are more quickly absorbed than plain water.

Start your activity early in the morning or in the evening for the coolest times. Cut your amount of exercise to 50 or 60 percent and work up over several weeks to your full time and effort.

Wear clothes of light-colored cotton. Don't change your clothes-- the wetness will help evaporation; dry clothes insulate you. Drop that towel--you need to be wet to get cool. Thinner people tolerate heat better than stout people.

If your pulse is even five to ten beats faster than usual, or if you feel as if you are working unusually hard, or if you are more breathless, **STOP.** Walk about in the shade, continue drinking, and **quit** the exercise. Avoid caffeine and alcohol; they are diuretics and will only cause you to lose more fluid. Seek medical help promptly if you don't get better within a few minutes.

If you live in a climate where the heat is extraordinary or the combination of heat and humidity is discouraging, then consider the ability of modern indoor exercise equipment to allow you to workout INSIDE and yet by video be OUTSIDE. On a hot, wet summer day you can be on your indoor cross-country ski machine in the Colorado mountains!

Most of the simple things described in this book can be done at home, at a health club, or in the mall, in a more controlled and comfortable enviomment.

ASTHMA AND CHRONIC OBSTRUCTIVE PULMONARY DISEASE

Rest used to be considered the most important part of the treatment for almost all your pulmonary problems. It is not so anymore. Regular activity can improve your effort tolerance. Walking, cycling, and stair climbing are equally effective. Your doctor can do studies of your breathing capacity and other studies to see if you have any heart limitations, and can determine your need for supplemental oxygen. "Breathing muscle" training and strengthening may be useful for you.

"Exercise induced asthma" is asthma brought on by a specific trigger--activity or exercise. It is primarily set off by airway cooling and drying, which brings on bronchospasm. There are several ways for you to avoid triggering that spasm. Avoid working out in very hot, dry areas or very cold, dry areas. Nasal breathing warms the air; a wet cloth placed over your nose and mouth in summer or a scarf over your nose and mouth in winter is helpful. During warm-up you may prevent triggering spasm with brief bursts of submaximal activity.

You will do best with water activities because they increase the moisture in the air.

Inhaled agents are very useful with rapid local activity, if you take them about 15 minutes before the activity. You may stop an attack already triggered with other inhalants.

VISIT OUR KITCHEN:
Activity Tools
In All Shapes And Sizes

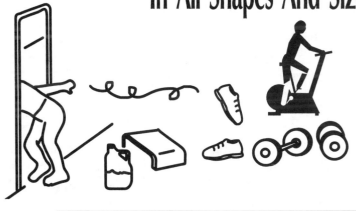

Chapter 11
Kitchen Gadgets/Little Helpers

Just the way modern kitchen gadgets help you whip up that gourmet meal with ease, so can some small pieces of apparatus help you prepare a safe and effective "à la carte" exercise stew. Some of these gadgets you will find in your house. Others, you will wish to buy. Gadgets can be very helpful. They will make your "cooking" more fun, so you will be more likely to continue to be active.

POTATO MASHERS

* **Free weights** can be purchased as cast-iron dumbells weighting two, five, eight, or ten pounds (usually they cost 50 cents per pound

and up, depending on covers, etc.). Use them as described in Chapter 12, or get instruction from a trainer. Soft weights of one to two pounds that fasten around your wrists or ankles are fine to use when you are not running or doing weight-shifting sports. A plastic gallon jug, when half filled with water, weighs four pounds (each pint of water is one pound).

You burn more calories when you walk carrying two- or three-pound weights. If your back is easily hurt, don't do this, because the weights may produce twisting strain as you walk. Ankle weights are all right if your back is good and you are only walking. Don't use ankle weights while jogging or running.

PANCAKES

* An **exercise mat** for abdominal curls and other floor exercises is comfortable. An old quilt, blanket, or mat for beach or pool works just as well.

WAFFLES

* **Shoes** for cross-training or courts are stiffer than shoes for jogging or running and are probably better for your purposes. SAS, Rockport, and Soft-Spot shoes are best for longer walking, especially if the terrain is rough or you must walk on hard cement surfaces. Aerobic workouts should be done on a carpet. If your feet are very flexible (flat, overpronated), you may need a well-padded arch support. Try one off the shelf first, but you may be better satisfied with a custom-made one. A health practitioner who deals with feet on a regular basis--such as an orthopedic surgeon or a podiatrist--will treat you best.

TEA TOWELS AND RAGS

* **Clothing** should be loose and comfortable but not sloppy. "Grunge" is popular--but don't get those floppy clothes caught in the machine. Colorful and cheerful wear is always helpful. Spandex is entirely wearer's choice, but it may feel and look good under looser shorts. Layering is important in colder seasons.

THERMOMETER--FEET

* **Pedometers** are useful, but read and follow the directions well. They can be used for shorter bites or to measure each day's cumula-

tive mileage. See if you really do "walk all day." Perhaps you are right! Aim for three to five miles over the course of the day if walking is your primary effort.

THERMOMETER--HEART

* **Pulse meters** are for the more serious exercise cook. The simpler ones that attach to finger or ear are accurate enough for most of us. For very serious cooks, there are "EKG" models that are extremely accurate because they transmit your heart's electrical impulse to your wrist monitor. They cost $85 to $125 or more.

STEAMER

* For a smooth and liquid diet, try the ever more popular **AQUAJOGGER.** It is a waistband of pretty flotation material that is very comfortable and safe; it allows you to tread water or run in water. You may do water calisthenics with your head up and your feet down, at your chosen level of effort. An informative booklet comes with this nice addition to your activity choices. Recently I have seen water paddles, water weights, and tethers that let you swim in place. (See Appendixes E and F for phone numbers and addresses.)

JELLO MOLD

* That **mini-trampoline** is wonderful for walking in place and bouncing a little, and it is very low impact. It is great for maintaining your balance and grace. A long time spent on it may irritate your knees, because it becomes saucer-shaped on impact.

Try one of the new **gel-filled seat covers** on your indoor or outdoor bike--they are great for tender bottoms.

TOO GOOD TO BE TRUE?

* True gadgets such as the Thigh-Master, Gut-Buster, and Abdominizer will help if used properly and according to directions. Motivators are always welcome. There are some reports of Gut-Busters coming apart and hurting folks, so be careful. There are other devices whose claims are so far unproven, such as the Mark II bust developer, the Astro-Trimmer exercise belt, and the Slim-Skins vacuum pants.

JUMPERS

* **Jump ropes** are for high-impact, high-intensity exercisers. If you were good at it when you were a kid, you can probably do it again if you start gently. You can make your own from heavy cord or wash line. The rope should reach from armpit to armpit while going under both feet. Put your palms up for twirling. Try it for 30 seconds with an easy two-step and then for 60 seconds jogging in place. Then repeat, if you can, several times. You need good shoes or a thick rug to absorb the impact.

SLIP AND SLIDE

* A new addition to kitchen gadgets that is inexpensive and easily tucked away is the **slideboard.** It can provide a good, gentle, low-impact sliding experience. But make no mistake--you can get a full-fledged aerobic workout with a slideboard, too. Most of them come with a video and instructions. No serious injuries are reported from slideboards yet, but some "lateral motion" strains of the hip, knee, or heel-cord are likely.

RECIPES

* Get a **USA map**, a big one, with stickers or pins. "GO" at 60 miles an hour and advance yourself a mile for each minute of exercise along whatever route you wish. Collecting daily minutes of activity or exercise will work well.

* Why not **travel the world?** "Fly" at jet speed, 500 miles per hour, and advance across oceans and continents at 8 miles per minute of exercise. Where shall we go?

* **Head phones** can help you concentrate wonderfully. The wired ones are cheaper. Infrared transmitted ones allow more freedom. The combination of a video exercise helper (audio and video) and earphones is total immersion, closer to "virtual reality."

* **Book racks** are helpful for long, not too bouncy or strenuous stationary bike rides. It is harder to maintain your target heart rate while reading. Some folks can use book racks on steppers.

DIGGING

* There are at least three sizes of **shovels**, and many types of blades. Get one you can lift when it is full of dirt. The handle should be long if there is not a cross-grip at the top. Get a long handle on your **hoe** also; short tools of all kinds can bend you over and make your back ache. A lightweight push mower may be just right for you to avoid that engine and be active too.

VISIT OUR KITCHEN

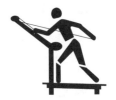

Chapter 12
Kitchen Appliances/For Serious Cooks

Before you invest in "major appliances" for your activity kitchen, be sure that you really want to be a serious cook. Although you may not need equipment that will be passed down from generation to generation, you will want good, sturdy tools that will encourage you to reach your goal of health and fitness.

Appliances differ from gadgets in that they are machines that simulate real activities. They can be marvelous additions to your life, or they can be harsh and painful taskmasters. I recommend that you try out various ones by renting them or using them in a health club before you buy. At least be sure that you can return the machine or trade it in if you can't make friends with it.

If your job is one that requires you to sit all day, you may wisely choose a stepper or treadmill or indoor skier. If you stand much of the time at work, a stationary bicycle may be perfect for you. So think about your own needs, and **"exercise à la carte."**

The PAR-Q (Physical Activity Readiness Questionnaire) is in Appendix G. Heart rates are discussed in Chapter 9 and Appendix M. Rate of perceived exertion (RPE) is discussed in Chapter 9 also. Please review these before you tackle an entrée.

MIXERS

Stationary Bicycles
* *May come without arm levers
  May come with only arm levers

May come with fixed arm levers
May come with detachable arm levers

* **Bicycle stands** with wind trainers or rollers let you mount your bicycle on a frame and ride it indoors.

* **Interactive** bicycles let tension be controlled by the rider and come with a video, a built-in computer program, a measure of the rider's heart rate, or some combination of these.

* **Recumbent** stationary bicycles are reported to lower the stress on painful backs and knees and be less prone to elevate blood pressure.

You need a sturdy bike that doesn't rattle when you shake it or climb on it. The seat needs to be comfortable. There should be wheels at one end so you can roll it, since most are very heavy.

Your stationary bike should be free-wheeling, so that as you stop pedaling, the pedals stop too, even if the flywheel continues to revolve. The seat and handlebars need to be adjustable. The instruction booklet should contain lots of helpful details.

You should be able to tilt the seat up in front just a little so you don't wear yourself out pushing yourself back on the seat. The seat should be adjusted high enough to leave your down leg bent just a little at the knee. Too high will cause you to rock back and forth and wear out your bottom. Speaking of which, look out for shorts with seams in the wrong places. There are sheepskin and gel-filled seat covers that are very welcome. The handlebars should let you sit forward comfortably, bent just a little, and should be padded or able to be padded. Use a fan to lend realism and to cool you off.

Try several bikes out for at least five minutes in a store, at a club, or at a friend's home. Buy one with your credit card and make sure you can return it if you find problems with you or it. Price range? Anywhere from $60 to $3,500.

With your stationary bike you need an easy adjustment for the flywheel tension; an odometer for the miles you travel; a speedometer; and a timer with a bell. There are lots of bells and whistles on the most expensive bicycles--they are there to add realism, provide information, and help you avoid boredom. You probably need a bicycle costing $300 to $750 for reasonably serious work. It is astonishing what you can buy at a garage sale.

The only wireless <u>interactive</u> bicycle is sold by IMPEX. The bike is controlled by a specially encoded video in your TV/VCR, so the feeling of hills and dales is very real. (See Appendix F for the address.) There are other bikes rigged so that you can play video games while you exercise!

Climb on the bike, start with low tension, at 40 to 50 revolutions per minute (RPM)--count on the upstroke--and pedal for 5 to 10 minutes if you are in pretty poor condition. Add more time and increase RPM and tension depending on your health. Be guided safely by your target heart rate zone (see Chapter 9.)

Read the booklet that comes with that bicycle!

Bicycle stands, or trainers, are stands to which you may clamp your outdoor bike, including hybrid or even mountain bikes, and make yourself ready for the good weather. They can be found at most bicycle specialty stores and at larger sporting goods stores. They offer a superb and inexpensive way to use your own bike as an exercise bike. Most stands cost less than $100 to $150. Some require you to remove the front wheel, which is easy. I like the ones that allow you to leave the front wheel on; the "steering" lends a bit of realism.

As you pedal you turn small rotary fans that increase resistance automatically as you increase speed. Some are controlled electromagnetically, which in the future will more easily allow interactivity to be part of the system.

Rollers provide a framework on which an outdoor bike may be ridden freely, in place, indoors. They are quite difficult and require lots of practice. They provide serious realism!

The feeling of riding a stationary bike and the skills required to ride a bike outdoors or on rollers are quite different. The main things missing from stationary bicycling are the balance and strength required outdoors. Training indoors can certainly increase your strength and aerobic conditioning.

MASHERS

Steppers and Stair Climbers
   *Moving stairs (escalator "down")
   *Steps that <u>YOU</u> move
      Alternately
      Independently
   *Vertical climbers for arms and legs
   *Interactive--step tension changes with terrain on a specially encoded video or with a program built into the climbing machine.

You need to try these machines out for several minutes in the store or somewhere, perhaps in a health club. They are very popular, so you may have to wait in line. If they are flimsy, you will constantly be worried about slipping off. It is best if the pedals are big and flat and stay that way. The pedals may be linked so that as one goes up the other goes down, but as your skills improve you will be more comfortable if the pedals operate independently. Comfort costs more. The resistance of the pedals may be controlled by air, fluid, or electromagnetism. You will like the feel of air-controlled or electromagnetically controlled pedals best. The vertical climbers require you to use both arms and legs and simulate rock climbing a little.

Start carefully with a short exercise time, short steps, and a slower pace, if possible. Use the rails for balance only--don't clutch them with a death grip to ease the weight on your feet. Keep your whole foot on the pedal, not just the ball of the foot. The odd feeling comes from never touching the ground; you never really get the feeling of pushing off. Think about stepping up, not down. But what a workout! Your pulse can rocket up to and beyond your target heart rate before you know it. A great workout in 13 minutes. Great for calves and buttocks (gluteal muscles).

Read the booklet!

PERCOLATOR

Treadmill
  *Motorized
  * Nonmotorized
  *Motorized
      Interactive
  *Poles for arms

Eighty-five percent of all treadmills sold are used for walking. They are coming down in price and going up in quality. Get one that has variable speeds at least up to eight miles per hour and a variable incline (0 to 8 percent). You will like it better if these variables can be controlled from the panel. You will need a wide surface that is long enough for your longest stride. If you are stout and or are going to run on it, you need a good strong treadmill with a good strong motor, or it will lag at each foot strike. A direct current (DC) motor is said to provide more even power.

At least one sturdy hand rail is important, and there should be enough foot room on both sides of the belt to let you stand off the belt when starting the machine. A reassuring feature is a safety strap to a switch that turns the machine off if you fall.

The recent addition of arm poles to some treadmills permits you to increase the number of muscles you use and the energy and fuel you spend per unit of time.

The least expensive type of treadmill uses you for the motor. In the past these have been very flimsy and hard to work. The newer models with a flywheel are much more secure, and some have poles or ropes and pulleys so your arms can work too--cross-training again. Soon there will be videos that will automatically, without wires, control speed and incline in keeping with the view on a screen. There are built-in computer programs to change speed and incline now. Treadmills are really looking good!

If the treadmill is your appliance of choice, dress as if you were really going walking and approach it with a program you would have in mind for walking. As you walk along, have a little bit of incline. Start with five minutes twice daily and add one or two minutes to each walk every week. (See the segment on walking in Chapter 4.)

Read the booklet! (Did I say that before?)

WASHER

Rowing Machines
  *Flywheels
  *Plungers
  *Interactive

This hard worker makes you use all your muscle groups. There are many ingenious arrangements for providing resistance. The hydraulic arms provide a satisfactory workout at a lower price. The flywheel models, especially those with a "fan-wheel," offer much more realism. Rowing machines may aggravate certain back problems. Ask your doctor or be sure you can return the machine. Maybe you could rent or borrow one or try one in a club for a month before buying an expensive one. There are rowers with a TV screen and graphics to provide a rowing companion and racing motivation.

Be sure to aim your arm pull stroke toward your belly, not toward your chin. Your legs provide the power, not your back. Put your arms forward before bending your knees.

READ the booklet!

DRYER

Tanning cabinets

It doesn't really matter whether a tanning cabinet provides light in the form of ultraviolet A (UVA) or ultraviolet B (UVB). Both are harmful--UVB more so than UVA. They are less harmful in smaller doses. It may seem self-defeating, and it is more expensive because it will take more sessions, but use a sunscreen with an SPF (sun protective factor) of 15 so that you tan much more slowly. This probably allows the cells in your skin (melanophores) to enlarge to produce the tan with less damage. Tanning salons are not very well regulated, nor are their machines always carefully calibrated. It doesn't matter much, since all UV light is harmful, but you don't want an overdose.

The same applies to tanning from the sun, too. Actually, 20 minutes of direct sunlight on just your hands and face or arms (one-tenth of your body's surface) will produce the daily amount of natural vitamin D you need to digest and process calcium into bone. You can get that during your walk or with a tanning machine. After that 20 minutes of useful exposure, use sunscreen of at least SPF 15 and wear a hat or protective clothing from ten o'clock to two o'clock.

Tumbling

Toning tables are one of the frauds of the health market that have had a flare of popularity and are still being relied upon by a surprising number of us. We would love to have exercise done for us as a passive thing. It seems to be the ideal way into activity and exercise. The only thing better would be to have a magic pill. Unfortunately, no such passive motion or magic pill does us the slightest bit of good. Toning tables, sadly, are not at all helpful in any activity plan. Perhaps they will entice some folks into a fitness place and lead them to real exercise.

Electronic muscle stimulation is a useful technique in rehabilitation and will help restore some bulk under certain conditions. However, normal nerves stimulating normal muscles are so much more superior in building muscle fibers that outside electrical stimulation

KNEADER

Ski machines
* Cross-country ski simulators
    Cords for arms
    Levers or poles for arms
    Flywheels
    Interactive
* Alpine ski simulators
    Lateral motion exercisers
    Simple arcs of motion
    Complex arcs of motion

Ski machines will really get you "cooking" in style. They offer the best aerobic challenge of all the appliances described in this chapter--and they offer it with very low impact. They work the most muscle groups. Those with cords rather than poles require a little more agility, coordination, and grace but will give you a harder workout.

Some models allow independent arm and leg motion; others require synchronization. Those with poles are more easily learned and are just as satisfactory. They are a bit less expensive. There are some very cheap and flimsy popular models.

Yours should cost $300 to $750. The most expensive ($1,500 or more) will last several generations at many miles per day.

Indoor cross-country ski machines simulate the outdoor sport. I am told by some that although the transfer of strength, skill, and grace may not be complete, these machines are a great help in getting ready for outdoor Nordic skiing.

Interactive videos that change the tension to match the ski terrain in specially designed indoor ski machines are available from Fitness Master dealers and from Nordic Track.

There also are lateral motion frames that simulate downhill skiing. The slideboards mentioned in Chapters 4 and 11 use lateral motion too.

There are several downhill or Alpine ski simulators on the market. Try these before you buy. Some are simple and some are very complex, expensive, and require lots of skill to use.

BIG KETTLES

Every kitchen needs a big kettle and several small ones!

Weight Lifting
* Fixed Machines
    Universal, Nautilus, Bow-Flex, Nordic Chair, Cybex, others
* All in one
    NordicFlex Gold, Solo Flex, Health-Max, Tri-Max, many others
* Weight bench
    Safety devices
* Free weights
    Dumbbells, barbells, hand weights

Health and fitness folks stress that any activity or routine should include both an aerobic element and a strengthening and endurance element. During aerobic activity, the larger muscles of your legs and hips are working to return blood to your heart, which raises its demand during exercise. The work encourages your heart to beat faster and your lungs to breathe faster--which provides the aerobic, oxygen-using part of your activity. Those large muscles act as if they were your "second heart." But while your leg and hip muscles are getting stronger, not much is happening to the muscles in your abdomen or upper body.

Abdominal curls can provide lower trunk strength because most of your front, or abdominal, muscles are, in fact, your back muscles. Think of your trunk as a barrel--all the "staves and hoops" need to be strong.

Your arms and shoulders need special attention, as well as your large back and chest muscles. It is for these muscles that resistance and strength training is really helpful.

The resistance in weight-lifting machines is usually provided by stacks of weights that the machine "holds" for you and allows you to lift safely (this is isotonic exercise).* Some of the more complex machines vary the resistance required throughout the arc of motion (for isokinetic exercise), much as your body does naturally.

---

* Isometric, isotonic, and isokinetic refer to three ways that muscles, joints, and forces work and can be exercised. The important thing is that in resistance exercising we are asking the muscles to do MORE work than usual, progressively, and that is what makes them larger and stronger.
    Isometric = Muscle working, joint still, force static
    Isotonic   = Muscle working, joint working, force static
    Isokinetic = Muscle working, joint working, force variable

chines vary the resistance required throughout the arc of motion (for isokinetic exercise), much as your body does naturally.

When you are shopping for a mini-gym, look for a sturdy frame with secure padding on the bench and on the weights. The cables should be strong and smooth running and require little snapping and unsnapping. Mini-gyms may not be suitable for very large or very small folks.

There are other methods of providing resistance: with movable elastic bands; with flexible rods of strong, light, composite material; with air pistons; or with hydraulic mechanisms.

Free weights are less expensive than weight-lifting machines and can be put away after use. All planes of motion, including "on your head," are possible with free weights. For well under $100 you should be able to get dumbells of two, five, and eight pounds, a rack for them, and a floor mat. (See the trial program described below.)

If you want to try free weights, it is probably best to invest in a consultation at a health club about a program especially for you. You can hurt yourself with free weights if you don't learn to use proper form in each exercise. Also, a club can offer individual and ongoing help as your skills advance. You might just like a health club setting best of all, so try it out. Maybe you can get a trial membership. There is no reason why you can't do activity and exercise both at home and at a club--they are equally effective in helping you.

COMBINATION MACHINES

There are many inventive folks who have put together hybrid exercise machines of an almost infinite variety. You will find weight benches and mini-gyms with a stepper at one end, treadmills with arm exercising poles, steppers with arm poles, bicycles with arm exercisers, dance and twist, chairs with built-in ropes and weights, and bicycles that come with a stand to use indoors or out. The combinations are limited only by an inventor's imagination. Try them first to be sure the one you might buy has the attributes you want.

TRIAL FREE-WEIGHT PROGRAM FOR BEGINNERS

Did you know that you still have almost all the muscle fibers that came with you? You do lose a few percent with aging. Each fiber is larger or smaller than it used to be. If it is larger, you are in "good shape" and strong. If the fibers are small and thin, you have been neglecting them. You can make the fibers larger and yourself stronger by using them. Muscle does <u>not</u> turn into fat.

For each free-weight exercise you want to do, find out how much weight you can easily lift ten times (each time is called a <u>repetition</u>). I found that for most exercises, two pounds seemed enough for the first week--especially in overhead lifts! I was pleasantly surprised at how rapidly I could increase the number of repetitions, and then I slowly increased the weights. Within three weeks I noticed an increase in my strength! Be sure you don't do free-weight exercises more often than every other day. Muscle tissue takes <u>24 to 48 hours</u> to repair and grow--and maybe a day longer in older folks.

Start with two or more pounds of weight in each hand. The variables of weight training are <u>pounds of weight</u> (2, 5, 8, 10, or more), <u>repetitions</u> performed (8 to 12), and number of <u>sets</u> of repetitions (1 to 3). It is best to start with light weights and modest numbers of repetitions. When the work gets too easy, go on to the next level.

Biceps: Sit, stand, or kneel with a dumbell or weight in each hand, your arms hanging down by your sides. Slowly curl one weight up as far as possible, in 2 to 4 seconds, then slowly lower it for 3 to 5 seconds. Repeat with the other arm, and continue alternately. Do 8 to 12 repetitions. Later work up to 2 or 3 sets.

Shoulders: Stand or sit with a dumbell in each hand and your arms straight down. Raise one up and forward to shoulder level, palm down. Hold briefly. Lower slowly. Alternate arms. Do 8 to 12 reps, and later increase to 2 or 3 sets.

Trapezius (neck/shoulder): Stand with your head straight. Put your chin down a little. Hold a dumbell in each hand. Lift your shoulders as if you were trying to touch your ears. Hold them up briefly. Lower them slowly. Do 8 to 12 repetitions. Later do 2 to 3 sets.

Now you have the idea. You can work overhead, or with your elbows bent and arms rotating, or in any number of positions. Be careful: use lighter weights whenever you start a new position.

These same admonitions and suggestions can be applied to the fixed-weight machines described above. These weights--fixed, padded, and safely controlled--might be more appropriate for a beginner or an older person.

TRY US, YOU'LL LIKE US:
Flavorful Motivators

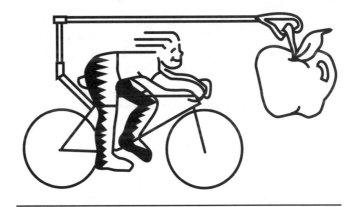

Chapter 13
Stimulants/Condiments

The big hurdle in activity is boredom. Outdoor activity is usually stimulating enough to keep you interested, but even then, music can be helpful. The immensely popular Sony Audio Walkman apparatus is clear evidence of this.

Indoor activities, on the other hand, require your ingenuity to provide motivation and diversion. From simply turning on the radio or the CD, tape, or record player for stimulating music to the complex "virtual reality" systems of the Air Force Trainer, the ingredients SENSORY FEEDBACK and SENSORY ENHANCEMENT are welcome indeed!

Many inventive motivational sensory stimulators are available and can be used by you at home right now. The ones chosen most often are video and audio helpers.

VIDEOTAPES

* Aerobic exercise videos

There are hundreds of exercise tapes, of all sorts. Next time you rent a video, ask about the exercise section and go look at some. Blockbuster has an good selection. Most are clearly marked. Start with a beginner's edition. Rent before buying: you may or may not like the people, the music, or the instruction. Occasionally, your library will have them. Jazzercise has been in business for 23 years, did you know that? They have produced a fine beginner's tape.

Any video should remind you about safety and seeing your doctor, list the instructor's credentials, and offer warm-up and cool-down periods. The program should offer various levels of difficulty. Look for simple, clear movements. You should be told early which motions are not as safe as others. Someone should state the goals for you and for the video tape.

Some exercises are just naturally done better indoors or in private, such as stretching or upper body, lower back, and pelvic tilt exercises. New dance routines are grand indoors, especially on a nasty rotten day. Videotapes can help you fill in missing parts in your activity, such as aerobics, strengthening, or yogalike stretch-and-relax. J. S. Missett of Jazzercise recently produced a home "circuit training" tape.

The most important guide is your own common sense in starting easily and advancing slowly.

* Age-Related Exercise Videos

Dancing Grannies, Richard Simmons's "Sweatin' to the Oldies" (he also has a beginner's tape), Angela Lansbury's "Positive Moves," and many others speak to the mature folks. Over 50? Try "More Alive," by Jo Murphy (MAC, P.O. Box 31872, Aurora, CO, 80041).

For Kids? Ages 5 to 12. "Hip Hop Animal Rock," by Gilda Marx, has good recommendations.

* Problem- or Condition-Related Exercise Videos

"Arthritis PACE" (People with Arthritis Can Exercise), from the Arthritis Foundation; "Back Health," from Joanie Greggains; "Wheelchair" and others for disabled people, from National Handicapped Sports; "Aerobics for Asthmatics," by gold medalist Nancy Hogshead (see Appendix F for address).

Covert Bailey's "Fit or Fat" video collection from PBS is a superb way to get educated, entertained, and motivated. Get his single video first--rent it if you can--to be sure you like his wonderfully unique style. Susan Powter's "Stop the Insanity" enthusiasm is also very engaging.

* Point-of-View Videos

These videos are made as if you were bicycling, skiing, walking, hiking, or climbing, and are to be used with the appropriate exercise machine. They lend realism and encouragement to your efforts. VIDEOCYCLE, NORDIC VISION, VIDEOHIKER, VIDEOSTRIDE, VIDEOSKIER, and others made for rowing are all available. They go into your VCR and play on your TV. Watch while you exercise! See Appendix C for phone numbers.

Motivating videotapes don't have to be complex. Pick a favorite travel or scenic video and turn the sound down. Then play the kind of stimulating music you like and have the best of "à la carte" choices!

* Alternative Exercise Videos

Videos showing you how to do t'ai chi ch'uan (both short and long forms), yoga, and many of the variations discussed in Chapter 7 can be found in video stores or in exercise video catalogues. (Call for the "YES! Bookshop and Video Catalogue" listed in Appendix C.)

* How-To, Skill-Related Exercise Videos

"Stretching" with Bob Anderson; "Gym Dandy" (comes with rubber tubing); and videos on weight training, nutrition, golf (there are several hundred of these), and skiing--both cross-country and downhill.

In fact, there are now videos to assist you in learning almost all the major sports of the world, from the complete novice level to the most advanced. Sybervision produces some unique teaching tapes for learning a sport.

* Exercise Video Catalogues (Appendix C)

See especially "The Complete Guide to Exercise Video," free from Collage Video, which contains very clear and honest descriptions of hundreds of videos. Personal help is available by phone! Browse the appendixes to this book for an amazing array of catalogues and information!

AUDIOTAPES

Loud, fast music makes us eat more and remarkably faster. Music has profound effects and can also make us work faster or slower. Our perception of activity changes a lot depending on what sort of music accompanies it.

Beats per minute may be important, but whatever you like and moves you is the right music: **"exercise à la carte."**

Music has been produced from new and old favorites, with rhythms built in, to be helpful in any activity or exercise--whether raking, mowing, sweeping, or walking.

When you use music while you walk, use these guidelines:

Miles per hour	Music beats per minute
3.0	105
3.5	120
4.0	135
4.5	150
5.0	160

* **Music:** Jazz, rock, classical--all have a role to play and someone who loves them.

* **Motivating audiotapes and CDs** have been produced with exercise machines in mind, such as stationary bicycles, indoor skiers, walkers, runners (treadmills), and steppers.

***Books** on tape

***Instructional lessons** of all sorts. Learn a foreign language while you get fit!

***Music catalogues** (see Appendix C).

BOOKS AND PRINT

An astonishing array of printed material is available to help you learn about the marvelous benefits of a healthy, fit life. ENJOY!

I found these especially useful; details are in Appendixes A through F:

* <u>Wellness Encyclopedia,</u> University of California at Berkeley.
* <u>Health Letters</u>
* <u>Home Fitness Journal,</u> CVT Productions, Inc.
* <u>Exercise for Health.</u> American Physical Therapy Association.
* <u>The Family Fitness Handbook.</u> Games for all.
* Dean Ornish, M.D., <u>Eat More, Weigh Less.</u>
* <u>Pep Up Your Life,</u> AARP.
* Covert Bailey, <u>The New Fit or Fat.</u>
* Magazines: <u>Self, Shape, Men's Health, American Health, The Physician and Sportsmedicine, Weight Watcher's Magazine.</u>
* <u>Keys to Fitness over Fifty.</u>
* <u>ACSM Fitness Book,</u> American College of Sports Medicine.
* Don R. Powell, Ph.D., <u>A Year of Health Hints.</u>

MISCELLANEOUS HELPERS
(and see Chapter 11, Kitchen Gadgets)

Fans. Use stationary or oscillating ones, for cooling. They may come as part of the resistance mechanism, especially in bikes, rowers, and steppers.

Earphones. From TV or tape player, wired or infrared transmitted.

Video transmitter. From one main VCR to a second TV in another room, which could be in front of your exercise area or machine. (Rabbit-Gemini, at Radio Shack.)

Water. AQUAJOGGER and other water workout gear. Belts to allow swimming in place.

Bicycle accessories. Seat covers, reading racks, padding for handlebars.

Jump rope. Elastic bands. Free weights with soft covers.

Computer programs. One called "Exercise Break" offers moving graphic stretches at your work station.

TRY US, YOU'LL LIKE US:

Chapter 14
Whetting Your Appetite/Staying Hungry

The spirit is willing but the flesh is weak.

In a recent survey by the National Sporting Goods Association, 50 percent of Americans said they were interested in being more active and yet had been unsuccessful in either starting or continuing any increased activity program! Another twenty-five percent were totally uninterested in any activity, and 25 percent were already engaged in some kind of activity or aerobic exercise.

If this paragraph sounds familiar, that's good! It was, and is, the opening statement and central theme of this book!

When your appetite for activity or exercise is lagging or you are just not hungry for it at all, a bit of spice and change is welcome motivation. Try adding some of these "condiments" to your dishes!

* Getting to the table to start is the first and most critical effort. The time, inclination, and motivation must all be present. So pick something active you <u>like</u> to do and do it, even if only a few minutes each day. Look at the suggestions in the earlier chapters of this "exercise à la carte" menu and you will surely find something your soul and body will welcome. Try the appetizers in Chapter 2, or the snacks in Chapter 3.

* After you have started, you will probably be fine for the first few days or even weeks, if you don't overdo it. Then you must vary your activity so your brain doesn't get bored or your body too painful.

You may get a little tired at first, but stay with it unless you are exhausted for an hour or so, or if your muscles and joints stay sore for more than two hours after exercise. If so, cut back--you are doing too much.

The most critical milestone seems to come at about six weeks, when the initial flush of success is wearing off and the "Is this all there is?" syndrome comes along. That is a good time to reward yourself. Find a friend to join you for a while. Consider your "investment to date" in sweat and equipment. More variability at about this time in your activity efforts often pays off in renewed physical and mental resolve. Are stimulants needed? Try Chapter 13.

Award yourself a bright new shirt or shorts for every one inch or five pounds lost. Concert tickets for 20 pounds.

* "Staying the course" is an old but useful expression--the course is your lifetime! You may provide your body and mind with extraordinarily rich and varied activity or with a set daily measure of fuel burned in exercises. Either course is fine--you can even alternate them. Whatever works--"exercise à la carte."

If you do nothing active for as short a time as three weeks, you must be careful not to jump back into activity at your previous high level. Your muscles will complain--they think you have retired them. Don't despair, just begin at one-half the effort and work up again.

* An increase in activity any time during your life will yield great benefits for the whole rest of it. Exercise probably does increase your life expectancy, at least a little, and it certainly will help to crowd all the worst of it into the very last of it! A recent study of 90-year-old folks showed that simple thigh exercises could increase strength by 200 percent in just a few weeks. This meant they were less likely to fall and break a hip. What a payoff!

* <u>Men's Health</u> magazine suggests that you "put your money where your mouth is" and bet your partner at least $40 that you will complete a two-month program (for example). Odds are high that both of you will.

* Speaking of numbers, count backward when doing repetitions. Makes them seem like less and less instead of more and more!

* Make an appointment, a contract, with yourself. Treat each activity appointment as importantly as you would a business meeting or a critical luncheon date.

* To get help in overcoming bad weather challenges, see Chapter

9. Visit the "kitchen gadgets" in Chapter 11.

* A jogging stroller can be used for walking too. It will help your whole family spend more time together; your mate can help with child care, too.

* Remember, you get full exercise credit for an enthusiastic evening spent line dancing at the Sundance Saloon, ballroom dancing at the Blue Moon, or rocking at JJ's. Your companion and best friend will love you for it.

* That "down" feeling about three o'clock in the afternoon can be quickly reversed by a brisk five-minute walk, especially with a friend. Perhaps that friend will be your "activity partner," and you can encourage each other from day to day to keep each other active.

* Avoid staleness by cross-training and alternating days. Take rest days. Avoid asking for too much. Try seasonal switching of programs. Learn to relax (see Chapter 15, Mellow Pleasures).

* Arrange frequent changes of music. You will use different muscles! There is music available with a variety of beats per minute in almost any style you can wish (see Chapter 13 and Appendix C). Try classical music sometimes, especially in stereo, with headphones. Exercise to MTV.

* Pedal your stationary bike backward, or sit backward on it while pedaling. It can be interesting. Walking backward down an ordinary staircase uses entirely different muscles than walking forward. It does require new balancing acts. Using your stepper backward increases thigh muscle use.

* Videotapes, either travel or scenic, are available to bring realism to your exercise machines. Point-of-view videos will be your companions on your exercise bicycle, stepper, stair climber, indoor ski machine, or treadmill. Some recent videos even interact with you and your machine to raise the level of realism to new heights (see Chapter 13 and Appendix C). If the music on them isn't hot enough, turn down the sound and turn on your own kind of music--then "exercise à la carte"!

* You have 168 hours available in each week.

    56 hours will be spent sleeping.
    40 will be spent at work.
    14 will be spent in the car.
    About 10.5 hours will be spent eating.

In front of the TV? <u>14 hours.</u>

That leaves 33.5 hours.

How about investing 30 minutes each day in ACTIVITY?!

YOUR DOCTOR AND PHYSICAL ACTIVITY RECOMMENDATIONS

The form in Appendix O was developed by a group under the leadership of the New Mexico Governor's Council on Health, Physical Fitness, and Sports and of the Greater Albuquerque Medical Association.

It was then mailed to the 1,150 M.D. members of the association, along with a poster to be put in their waiting rooms inviting their patients to ask them about personal activity.

The form in Appendix O is for you to copy, if you wish, and take to your doctor. Take a copy of the letter too. Ask for his or her specific comments on your activity, because he or she will know about your needs and limitations and can advise you. Look it over and pencil in your own thoughts before you ask for your doctor's.

ON THE SOFA, LATER:
Body, Mind and Spirit

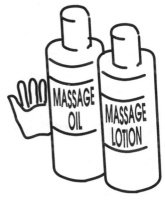

Chapter 15
Mellow Pleasures/The Right Tools

A gentle massage, a few minutes of quiet, deep breathing in the middle of a hectic day, a good belly laugh--all these mellow pleasures will help reduce stress, and reducing stress is vital to your good health. They just plain feel wonderful, too!

MASSAGE

Massage is one of oldest therapies in the history of humankind. Surprisingly, little is known about it in a scientific way. Its recipients know that through massage, muscles can be relaxed, mental stress eased, muscle pains and spasms relieved, and probably blood flow increased to skin and muscle.

One of the techniques common in America is Swedish massage, which is a gentle stroking and kneading and may include percussive hand use. Another is acupressure (shiatsu), which is becoming more popular and involves firmer, more static pressure on the skin and underlying tissues. Since 1980, warm-water immersion massage has exploded in popularity; it is called <u>watsu.</u>

Light oils with or without scent are helpful in avoiding too much friction, and they feel wonderful. Almond, sesame, and coconut oils are available in health food stores. Warm the oils to aid lubrication and communication.

Do not massage acute injuries--find out what has been injured first by consulting your doctor or medical partner. "Rest, Ice, Compress, and Elevate": this combination is called the RICE approach to acute injuries.

Contact the American Massage Therapy Association (AMTA) at 708-864-0123 for a list of members around you.

Massage for one . . . Start out with a nice warm bath or shower. Use a good body oil and then . . . Begin at your feet and pull each toe in turn, then slowly bend all your toes together. Grasp your foot, place both thumbs on the sole, and gently make rotations. An old-fashioned Coke bottle makes a great roller--not too hard. Work your way up the calves; massage toward your heart.

Your neck loves massage; use your fingertips to knead the big trapezius muscle that runs from the base of your skull halfway down your back and out to the points of your shoulders on both sides. Near your skull, knead the same side of your body, and as you get down to your shoulders, use the opposite hand.

Massage for two . . . is very satisfactory whether the other one is a friend, a professional, or both. I suggest you treat yourself and a friend to a massage gift. You can take turns being taught by an instructor to massage each other. Then proceed to more advanced techniques.

When you do start on your own, I think your partner's back is probably the best place to begin. A pillow under the abdomen of the person lying prone will relieve any stress on his or her lower back. A folded towel under the forehead will keep the neck from twisting too much to the side.

Work the warm oil into your hands and then follow the contours of your partner's shoulder blades, massaging over the shoulders, then down the back near the spine, and gradually out over the ribs and down to the upper buttocks, which are often very tender. Be kind--ask your partner if the pressure is firm enough or too firm, and so forth. Books and videotapes offering massage instruction are available (see Appendix C).

RELAXATION TECHNIQUES

"If a string has one end, then it has another."

Don't miss out on one of the greatest aids to health and fitness ever conceived. It is the other end of the activity string ("strung-out" is not badly named). The ability to let down for just 10 or 15 minutes once or twice a day is vitally important to staying well.

The **simplest technique** is to sit down in a quiet place and breathe. Pretty wild? Lots of people go around holding their breath, full of tension, all day! Proper breathing is not shallow and fast; that is hyperventilation, and it continues your uptight feeling or, worse, it makes you feel dizzy and fall down. The trick is to take deep breaths from your abdomen. Put one hand on your chest and one on your stomach. Taking a slow deep breath through your nose, make your stomach go out but not your chest. It's easy, and you won't need to put your hands there very long to learn the feeling. Breathe out through your mouth. Not very fast. Gently. Even five minutes is very relaxing.

The **Jacobson Progressive Relaxation** technique prefers that you lie down. Tighten each group of muscles one at a time, and feel the tension increase for two to five seconds. Now let the muscles go limp and feel the relaxation. Think your way from head to toe. This method takes longer, but is well worth it.

Benson Relaxation Response suggests that you sit quietly, eyes closed. Relax your muscles beginning at the toes and breathe in through the nose, out through the mouth. Say one word over and over to empty your mind (this is called a *mantra*) for 10 to 15 minutes. Be passive. It will take some practice. Works wonders.

Guided imagery is a self-directed daydream over which you have complete control and in which you travel in great detail. Sit quietly, breathing properly. Think of a pleasant time, then see and feel as vividly as you can all the details--what, where, when, colors, people, seashore, mountains, smells, everything.

Laughing heartily about 50 times a day uses up about 100 calories and does ever so much good! It even is said to increase your immune response. Don't take yourself too seriously. The CEO of that fabulously successful company, Southwest Airlines, is constantly laughing and helping those around him to enjoy life. The flight attendants did, too, but were asked by the FAA to get serious.

"SMILE!" says Paul Ekman, Ph.D., psychologist at the University of California at San Francisco. Amazingly, whether it is spontaneous or forced, it stimulates happiness changes in your brain!

Have an end-of-the-day plan. Remember, "no matter where you go, there you are." If you are away from home, bring a piece of home with you for your room. Before you return home from work, try to sit quietly for a few minutes before connecting with all the folks who love and need you at the end of your busy day. They will appreciate it and so will you.

STRESS REDUCTION

Much of the preceding discussion has been about stress reduction, which really is essential to your health, if not to your fitness. Don't let your frantic desire to be <u>fit</u> increase your stress level. Sound strange? It isn't--ask the "obligatory runner" who can't function at all if he or she doesn't have that daily run.

Stressed out? Hypertension, irregular heartbeat, headaches, insomnia, appetite changes, fatigue, irritability, and poor concentration got the upper hand? All can be symptoms of, or added to by, tension and stress.

The main damage of constant stress is caused by a perfectly normal bodily reaction to threats. We are on a balance beam between "fight or flight." That is, we are keyed to run like hell or slug it out. The ancient threats of being eaten have been replaced by difficult situations over which we have equally little control. Our bodies have only the ancient reaction to help us, and when stress-related chemicals such as adrenalin hang around a long time, they damage us.

Your first need is to recognize that **you** are reacting, and then do something else about it. Much of the stress may come from within you, especially after a long time at it. Usually, you can control only you and not the external forces pushing on you, so start there. If you are as controlled as you can get, then approach the external threats.

Exercise and activity are natural relievers of the stress chemicals. They are the best thing by far that you can do toward lowering your body's reaction to threats. It is amazing how solutions will come to you while you are working your physical body--your brain can help more with good blood flow!

Don't forget that stress is a normal part of life itself and probably accounts for most of the real advances in civilization. By no means does all stress come from the workplace!

Family worries and job dissatisfaction can play a large role in pre-cipitating and aggravating physical symptoms such as neck, shoulder, arm, hand, and lower back pains.

Try some **Action Snacks** (Chapter 3), followed by a **Relaxation Technique** as outlined above.

GATHERING YOUR À LA CARTE MENU:
CUSTOMIZING YOUR PLAN

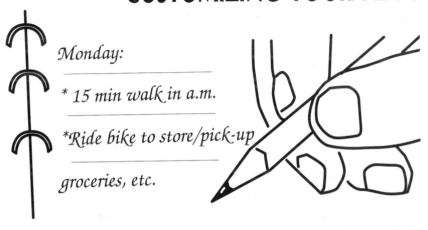

Monday:
_____
* 15 min walk in a.m.
_____
*Ride bike to store/pick-up
_____
groceries, etc.

Chapter 16
**Principles, Goals, Book Reviews and
Sample Menus**

**Before you actually pick a menu,
did you <u>really</u> look at the questions in the PAR-Q (Appendix G)?
If not, please do it now, so that you do not hurt you!**

The American College of Sports Medicine, the Centers for Disease Control, and the President's Council on Physical Fitness recently offered official exercise guidelines for **HEALTH;** these encourage you to "do your regular, everyday work tasks as you accumulate 30 minutes of enthusiastic, real activity on most days."

Standard guidelines for aerobic exercise from these highly respected groups have been, and remain, 20 to 60 minutes of aerobic workout three to five times a week, if your goal is improvement in **FITNESS**.

The new guidelines have to do with **HEALTH**, the previous ones with **HEALTH and FITNESS**. We talked about the differences in the introduction.

I suggest that you select from this activity/exercise menu those items that will let you accumulate 30 to 40 minutes of activity during each day, so that you use an extra 200 "activity calories." This is a way to measure what you are doing. In a surprisingly short time, you will easily "just do it" without keeping track of time or calories.

THINKING ABOUT GOALS

Activities	Description	Aerobic Effort
Couch potato	Sedentary	40 percent
Activities of daily living	Light work	50 percent
Regular exerciser	Medium work	60 percent
Chopping weeds or wood, mopping	Hard work	70 percent
Shoveling snow	Very hard work	80 percent
10K run or more	Prime fitness	

RECOMMENDED READING

**These are recently published books
on health and fitness which I recommend to you;
sources are in Appendix A.**

The American College of Sports Medicine, one of the foremost and most respected fitness organizations in the world, has produced the ACSM Fitness Book. It has wonderfully simple directions for measuring your present fitness level and advising you on advancing safely and steadily. A virtually perfect guide for the serious beginner.

The Wellness Guide to Lifelong Fitness, just off the presses as I write, is by the editors of the fine Wellness Letter from the University of California at Berkeley. Timothy White, Ph.D., and his coworkers have put together a book that is not only a photographic work of art but also contains all the words needed to understand why the well-demonstrated exercises are important. This is a book for the serious beginner, but it can carry you far beyond that into vitality, health, and fitness.

Living with Exercise is from the Cooper Institute for Aerobics Research in Dallas and is by Steven N. Blair, P.E.D., who must be an excellent communicator. The book takes the familiar form of a school workbook and is very nonthreatening. The words are simple, and Blair has a wonderful way of explaining complex subjects. It is about as interactive as a book can be. It is a starting-out kind of book for adults of all ages, but it reaches out to children and young people as well.

Fitness Without Exercise, by Bryant A. Stamford, Ph.D., and Porter Shimer, is a book I found after the first few drafts of mine were done. This is my same treatise, done scientifically and beautifully. I recommend it to you without hesitation for an easy-to-read but amazingly complete study of human energy expenditures. I am sure that at the time of its publication in 1990, Dr. Stamford was unpopular for his views that the most important human effort is natural work and that it is usually plenty for a long and healthy life!

The New Fit or Fat. The "old" one never left the scene, but Covert Bailey has revised this wonder book to make it even more user friendly! In concert with Bailey's other offerings, such as his book for women, the one with diets, and his wonderful videos from the PBS collection (see Appendix C), this unique and enjoyable presentation is very welcome.

The Exercise Exchange Program, by Dr. James M. Rippe with Patricia Amend (and recipes by Judy F. Pang), is essentially a cafeteria from which you may design your own diet and workouts. Rippe continues to add to his previous books to spread the word about life, health, mind, and activity. This is for the serious person who is already well organized and can choose and follow a pattern. All the pieces are here and need only construction.

Pep Up Your Life is the usual grand publication from the American Association of Retired Persons. It was prepared with the President's Council on Physical Fitness and Sports by Richard O. Keeler, Ph.D., and York Onnen, director of program development for the president's council. It just came to my desk, and let me tell you it is a fine, sensible, carefully measured approach to activity and exercise. Prepared for "mid-life and older persons," I could recommend it for ANYONE who might be starting activity from scratch. (See Appendix F for AARP's address.)

SAMPLE MENUS

The caloric figures in the sample menus that follow were gathered and interpolated from many sources, but especially from two books:

Fitness Without Exercise. Bryant Stamford, Ph.D., and Porter Shiner. Warner Books, New York. 1990.

The Exercise Exchange Program. Dr. James M. Rippe, with Patricia Amend. Simon and Schuster, New York. 1992.

SAMPLE: à la carte MENU

	Beginner	Light Work	Hard Work	Harder
MONDAY	Hang clothes outside (10 min.)	Scrub floor (10 min.)	Dig in garden (30 min.)	Jog (30 min.)
	30 calories	40	180	230
TUESDAY	Vacuum room (10 min.)	Rake leaves (15 min.)	Wash windows (20 min.)	Shovel snow (20 min.)
	30	50	90	200
WEDNESDAY	Weed garden (10 min.)	Swim (20 min.)	Climb stairs (5 times a day)	Run (30 min.)
	40	70	90	300
THURSDAY	Mop floor (10 min.)	Walk (15 min.)	RELAX	Bicycle in or out (40 min.)
	40	70		250
FRIDAY	Wash windows (10 ,min.)	Shop/ walk (30 min.)	Swimming aquatics (30 min.)	Walk (60 min.)
	40	100	120	360
SATURDAY	Dance (10 min.)	Chairs (10x3)	Bicycle in or out (20 min.)	Dance (60 min.)
	80	120	125	300+
SUNDAY	RELAX	Golf (2 hrs.)	Walk (30 min.)	RELAX
		320	180	

SAMPLE: à la carte MENU

	Beginner	Light Work	Hard Work	Harder
MONDAY	Walk bsiskly (5 min.)	Walk briskly (10 min.)	Walk 3.5 MPH (30 min.)	Walk 3.5 MPH (60 min.)
	30 calories	60	180	360
TUESDAY	10 Steps 2 times	Abd. curls (5), 2 lb. wts.	10 steps 4 times	abd. curls (10) 2-5 lb. wts.
	35	35	70	75
WEDNESDAY	Abd. curls (5)	Walk 10 min. Abd. curls (5)	Bike out or stationary (30 min.)	Walk 4.0 MPH (40 min.)
	20	80	225	330
THURSDAY	Arise from chair 5 times	10 steps 5 chairs	Abd. curls 10 5 lb. wts.	Bike out or stationary (45 min.)
	30	50	75	330
FRIDAY	Walk briskly (5 min.)	Bike, stationary (15 min.)	Walk or bike (30 min.)	REST
	30	110	200	
SATURDAY	2 lb. wts. Abd. curls (3)	Walk briskly (10 min.)	Chairs 10 2-5 lb. wts.	Abd. curl, 10 times 2 5-8 lb. wts.
	30	60	80	140
SUNDAY	Walk 5 min. with 2 lb.	Walk 10 min. with 2 lb.	REST	Walk 30 min.
	40	80		180

APPENDIXES

Appendix A

Books

ACSM Fitness Book. American College of Sports Medicine. Leisure Press, a division of Human Kinetics Publishers, Box 5076, Champaign, IL 61825-5076, 800-747-4457.

A Year of Health Hints. Don R. Powell, Ph.D. American Institute of Preventive Medicine. Rodale Press, Emmaus, PA, 313-352-7666. 1990.

Biomarkers: The 10 Keys for Prolonging Vitality. William J. Evans, Ph.D. Fireside Books, 1230 Ave. of the Americas, New York, NY 10020.

Consumer Reports Books. 800-272-0722.

Eat More, Weigh Less. Dean Ornish, M.D. Harper Collins Publishers, New York. 1993.

Family Fitness Handbook. Bob Glover and Jack Shepherd. Viking Penguin. 1989. Reprinted by Family Digest, Inc., 7002 W. Butler Pike, Ambler, PA 19002. 1994.

Fitness and Fallacies: Everyone's Guide. Rick De Lorme, M.A., M.S., and Fred Stransky, Ph.D. Kendall/Hunt Publishing Company, 2460 Kerper Blvd., P.O. Box 539, Dubuque, IA 52004-0539.

Fitness Without Exercise. Bryant Stamford, Ph.D., and Porter Shiner. Warner Books, New York. 1990.

Fitness the Dynamic Gardening Way. Jeffrey Restuccio. Balance of Nature Publishing. 800-507-2665.

Guidelines for Exercise Testing and Prescription. Fourth Edition. ACSM. Lea and Febiger, Philadelphia, PA, 215-251-2230. 1991.

Healing Back Pain. John Sarno, M.D. Warner Books, 1271 Ave. of the Americas, New York, NY 10020.

Healthy People 2000. U.S. Department of Health and Human Ser-

Keys to Fitness Over Fifty. Jo Murphy. Barron's Educational Series, Inc., 250 Wireless Blvd., Hauppauge, NY 11788.

Live Longer Cookbook. Reader's Digest Association, Inc., Pleasantville, NY. 1992.

*Living with Exercise. Steven Blair. American Health Publishing Company, Dallas, TX, 800-736-7323. 1991.

Minute Health Tips. Thomas G. Welch, M.D. DCI/CHRONIMED Publishing, P.O. Box 47945, Minneapolis, MN 55447-9727.

*Pep Up Your Life: A Fitness Book for Mid-Life and Older Persons. Richard O. Keeler, Ph.D., and York Onnen. Aided by the President's Council on Physical Fitness and Sports. AARP (American Association of Retired Persons). l994.

Sports Medicine. Otto Appenzeller, M.D., Ph.D., and Ruth Atkinson, M.D. Second Edition. Urban and Schwarzenverg, Baltimore. 1983.

*The Exercise Exchange Program. Dr. James M. Rippe, with Patricia Amend. Simon and Schuster, New York. 1992.

The Indoor Bicycling Fitness Program. Jane S. Peters. McGraw-Hill Book Company, New York. 1985.

The New Fitness Formula of the '90s. The National Exercise for Life Institute, Box 2000, Excelsior, MN 55331.

*The New Fit or Fat. Covert Bailey. Houghton Mifflin Company, P.O Box 230877, Tigard, OR 97223. 1991.

The Wellness Encyclopedia. University of California, Berkeley. Published by Houghton Mifflin Company, Boston, 800-829-9170. 1991.

*The Wellness Guide to Lifelong Fitness. Dr. Timothy White, Ph.D., and the editors of the *Wellness Letter.* University of California, Berkeley. REBUS, New York. Distributed by Random House. 1993.

30 Exercises for Better Golf. Frank W. Jobe, M.D., and Diane R. Schwab, M.S., R.P.T., with Bill Bruns. Champion Press, Inglewood, CA, 212-419-8669. 1986.

* Reviewed in Chapter 16.

Appendix B
Magazines and Periodicals

American Health. 800-365-5005

Arthritis Today. 800-283-7800

Bottom Line Personal. 800-274-5611

Cooking Light. 800-336-0125

Eating Well. 800-678-0541

Fitness. 800-888-1181

Health. 800-274-2522

Home Fitness Journal. 800-624-4952

Longevity. 800-333-2782

Men's Fitness. 800-998-0731

Men's Health. 800-666-2303

Prevention. 800-666-2503

Runner's World. 800-666-2828

Self. 800-274-6111

Shape. 800-998-0731

Successful Home Fitness. 800-624-4952

Walking Magazine. 800-678-0881

Weight Watcher's Magazine. 800-876-8441

Appendix C
Free Catalogues

"Covert Bailey's Products" 800-676-3263

"Collage Video." 800-433-6769

"Destination Fitness Workout Videos." Catalogue for point-of-view videos, music tapes, and compact discs for stationary cycling, ski machines, steppers, and treadmills. 800 624-4952

"Golf Smart" (videos). 800-637-3557

"Golf Videos Direct." 800-247-8273

Jazzercise catalogue. Tapes and information. 800-548-8927

"Nature Recordings." 800-228-5711

Nordic Track catalogue of products. 800-892-2174

"Self Care Catalogue." 800-345-3371

"Sybervision." 800-678-0887

"The Complete Guide to Exercise Videos." 800-433-6769

"Wellness Book" catalogue. 800-422-2320

"Workout Music." Sports Music Inc. 800-878-4764

"YES! Bookshop and Video Catalogue." Alternative motions. Personal awareness and "oneness." 800-937-1516.

Appendix D

Health Letters

Many of these health letters will send you a free sample before you subscribe, or will sell you an index of past issues.

Consumer Reports Health Letter. Consumer Reports, Subscription Dept., Box 52148, Boulder, CO 80322. 800-525-0643.

Consumer Reports on Health. Consumer's Union of the United States, Yonkers, NY 10703-1057. 800-234-2188.

Environmental Nutrition Newsletter. Environmental Nutrition, Inc., 2112 Broadway, New York, NY 10023. 212-362-0424.

Executive Health's Good Health Report. The Institute for Medical Information, 383 Rt. 46 W., Fairfield, NJ 07004. 800-935-0074.

Executive Fitness. Rodale Press, 33 E. Minor St., Emmaus, PA 18098. 212- 967-5171.

FitNews. American Running and Fitness Association, Bethesda, MD. 800-766-2372.

Harvard Medical School Health Letter. Harvard University, Department of Continuing Education, 79 Garden St., Cambridge, MA 02138. 617-495-5234.

Health Confidential. Box 53408, Boulder, CO 80322. 800-289-0409.

Healthline. The C. V. Mosby Co., 11830 Westling Industrial Dr., St. Louis, MO 63146. 314-872-8370.

Home Fitness Journal. CVT Productions, Inc., 440 Charnelton #220, Eugene, OR 97401. 800-624-4952.

John's Hopkins *Fitness Over 50.* P.O. Box 420176, Palm Coast, FL 32142.

John's Hopkins *Fitness Over 50*. P.O. Box 420176, Palm Coast, FL 32142.

Mayo Clinic Health Letter. The Mayo Clinic, 200 1st S.W., Rochester, MN 55905. 800-333-9038.

Men's Confidential Newsletter. P.O. Box 7315, Red Oak, IA 51591-0315. 800-666-2106.

Nutrition Forum. George F. Stickley Co., 210 W. Washington Square, Philadelphia, PA 19106. 215-546-2390.

People's Medical Society Newsletter. C/o the Society, 462 Walnut St., Allentown, PA 18102. 215-770-1670.

Running and FitNews. American Running and Fitness Association, 4405 East-West Highway, Suite 405, Bethesda, MD 20814. 800-766-ARFA.

Successful Home Fitness. CVT Productions, Inc., 440 Charnelton #220, Eugene, OR 97401. 800-624-4952

The Edell Health Letter. Hippocrates, Inc., 475 Gate Five Rd., Suite 100, Sausalito, CA 94965. 415-332-5866.

The Health Letter. Dr. Lawrence E. Lamb, c/o King Features Syndicate, 16 E. 45th St., New York, NY 10017. 800-526-5464.

Tufts University *Diet and Nutrition Letter*. P.O. Box 57857, Boulder, CO 80322-7857. 212-608-6516.

University of California at Berkeley *Wellness Letter*. P.O. Box 359148, Palm Coast, FL 32035. 800-829-9170.

University of Texas *Lifetime Health Letter*. P.O. Box 420342, Palm Coast, FL 32142-0342. 800-829-9177.

Appendix E

More Phone Numbers and Addresses

Aerobics and Fitness Foundation. 800-233-4886

American Academy of Orthopaedic Surgeons. 800-346-2267

American College of Sports Medicine. P.O. Box 1440, Indianapolis, IN 46206

American Council on Exercise. 800-529-8227

American Diabetes Association. 800-232-3472

American Heart Association. 800-242-8721

American Running and Fitness Association. 800-766-2372

American Self Help Clearing House. 201-625-7101

AQUAJOGGER 800-922-9544

Arthritis Foundation, Inc. 800-283-7800

"Exercise Break." Computer Program. Hopkins Technology, 421 Hazel Lane, Hopkins MN 55343. 612-931-9376

National Council on Aging. 800-424-9046

National Health Information Center. U.S. Department of Health and Human Services, Public Health Service. List of toll-free numbers. ODPHP National Health Information Center, P.O. Box 113, Washington, DC 20013-1133. 800-336-4797

National Handicapped Sports. 800-966-4647

NOSAD (National Organization for Seasonal Affective Disorders). P.O. Box 40133, Washington, DC 20016

Sybervision. 800-678-0887

The American Dietetic Hotline. 800-366-1655

The National Exercise for Life Institute. 800-358-3636

Women's Sports Foundation. 800-227-3988

YMCA of the USA. 800-872-9622

Appendix F

More Information of All Sorts

"Aerobics for Asthmatics." Gold medalist Nancy Hogshead. Video. Heinlyn Productions, 10301 Georgia, Silver Springs, MD 20902.

American Academy of Orthopaedic Surgeons. 6300 N. River Rd., Rosemont, IL 60018. 800-346-2267. Ask about their brochures: "Lift It Safe!" about preventing and treating back pain, and "Live It Safe," about avoiding and treating osteoporosis.

American Association of Retired Persons. 3200 E. Carson St., Lakewood, CA 90712. Exercise publication: *Pep Up Your Life.*

American College of Obstetricians and Gynecologists. Resource Center, 409 12th St. SW, Washington, DC 20024. Ask for a copy of "Exercise during Pregnancy and Postnatal Period" (home exercise programs), ACOG *Technical Bulletin* no. 189, February 1994.

American Council on Exercise. Information on starting exercise, weight control, and kid's fitness. 800-529-8227.

American Orthopaedic Foot and Ankle Society. How to, selection of sports shoes. Free brochure. 800-235-4855.

American Physical Therapy Association. 1111 Worth, Fairfax, VA 22314. SASE for free information on health topics.

Excel Sports Science. AQUAJOGGER and more. 800-922-9544.

"Healthy People 2000: Physical Activity Objectives." U.S. Department of Health and Human Services. SASE to HP2000 Objectives, c/o American College of Sports Medicine, P.O. Box 1440, Indianapolis, IN 46206-1440. (Also ask for "Exercise Lite.") For information, call 1-800-336-4797.

Impex Manufacturing. Interactive VideoCycle (IVC). 818-359-6868.

National Osteoporosis Foundation. 211 M St. NW, Washington, DC 20037.

"PALS: Personal Aerobics Lifestyle System." Self-assessment (mail back) guide. $22.50 from the Cooper Institute for Aerobics Research, 12330 Preston Road, Dallas, TX 75230-9990. 214-701-8001.

Pyramid food guide poster. **Free** from General Mills. 800-247-4393.

Rollerblade, Inc. Information. SASE envelope and $1 (MO or check) to:P.O. Box 59224, Dept P, Minneapolis, MN 55459. (Better Fitness, Michael O'Shea, Parade Magazine, 8/28/94)

"Safety for Older Americans." Booklet from the U.S. Consumer Product Safety Commission, Washington, DC. 20207. 800-638-2772.

"The Benefits of Regular Exercise." IRSA. Will send a list of health clubs. The Association of Quality Clubs, 253 Summer Street, Boston, MA 02210.

"The Food Guide Pyramid." U.S. Department of Agriculture, U.S. Department of Health and Human Services. 1992. Check or money order ($1.00) to Superintendent of Documents, U.S. Government Printing Office, Washington DC, 20402.

Wheat Foods Council. Suite 111, 5500 So. Quebec, Englewood, CO 80111. 303-694-5828.

Appendix G

PAR-Q: Physical Activity Readiness Questionnaire

Before beginning your exercise program, take this simple test. Answer the questions below. If there are <u>any</u> yes answers, postpone your exercise or fitness plans until you get medical consultation and clearance.

1. Has a doctor ever said that you have a heart condition and recommended only medically supervised activity?

2. Do you have chest pain brought on by physical activity?

3. Have you developed chest pain in the past month?

4. Do you tend to lose consciousness or fall over as a result of dizziness?

5. Do you have a bone or joint problem that could be aggravated by the proposed physical activity?

6. Has a doctor ever recommended medication for your blood pressure or for a heart condition?

7. Are you aware through your own experience, or through a doctor's advice, of any other physical reason against your exercising without medical supervision?

* If you answered **"NO"** to all questions accurately and honestly, you have reasonable assurance of your present suitability for a graduated exercise program.

* If you have a temporary minor illness, such as a common cold, postpone the beginning of your program.

There is NO guarantee that any protection from sudden death is afforded by ANY pre-test, even those more complex than PAR-Q.

Please refer to **Appendix O, Your Doctor Partner.**

Reference: "The Canadian Home Fitness Test: 1991 Update." R. J. Shephard, S. Thomas, and I. Weller. *Sports Medicine* 1, p. 359, 1991.

Appendix H

Food Guide Pyramid (see next page also)

The food guide pyramid tells you to eat a variety of foods each day:

6 - 11   servings from the bread, cereal, rice, and pasta group;
3 - 5   from the vegetable group;
2 - 3   from the fruit group;
2 - 3   from the milk, yogurt, and cheese group;
2 - 3   from the meat, poultry, fish, dry beans, eggs, and nuts group;
Sparingly from the fats, oils, and sweets group.

Everyone should have at least the smaller number of servings. Then if you need to eat more calories, have more food.

How much is a serving?

Bread, cereal, rice, and pasta: 1 slice bread; 1 ounce cereal; 1/2 cup cooked cereal, rice, or pasta.

Vegetables: 1 cup raw, leafy vegetables; 1/2 cup other vegetables (cooked or raw); 3/4 cup vegetable juice.

Fruit: 1 medium apple, banana, or orange; 1/2 cup chopped, cooked, or canned fruit; 3/4 cup fruit juice.

Milk, yogurt, and cheese: 1 cup milk or yogurt; 1-1/2 ounces natural cheese; 2 ounces process cheese.

Meat, poultry, fish, dry beans, eggs, and nuts: 2 - 3 ounces cooked lean meat, poultry, or fish; 1/2 cup cooked dry beans; 1 egg or two tablespoons peanut butter count as 1 ounce of meat.

Fats, oils, and sweets: Use as little as possible.

This information came from a Cheerios breakfast cereal box! **Isn't that grand?** You may call 800-247-4393 and get a food guide poster.

The Food Guide Pyramid

Key
- ● Fat (naturally occurring & added)
- ▼ Sugars (added)

These symbols show fat and added sugars in food. They come mostly from fats, oils, and sweet group. But foods in other groups-such as cheese or ice cream from the milk group or french fries from the vegetable group-can also provide fat and added sugars.

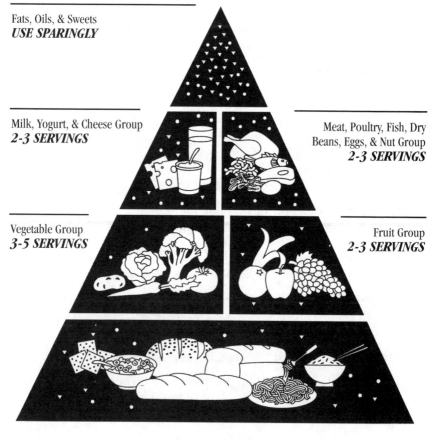

Fats, Oils, & Sweets
USE SPARINGLY

Milk, Yogurt, & Cheese Group
2-3 SERVINGS

Meat, Poultry, Fish, Dry
Beans, Eggs, & Nut Group
2-3 SERVINGS

Vegetable Group
3-5 SERVINGS

Fruit Group
2-3 SERVINGS

Bread, Cereal, Rice, & Pasta Group
6-11 SERVINGS

Source: USDA's Food Guide Pyramid booklet by Human Nutrition Information Service (HNIS)

Appendix I

Risk Factors for Osteoporosis. Calcium in Some Foods.

The more times you answer "yes" to these questions, the greater is your risk of developing osteoporosis.

1. Do you have a small, thin frame, or are you Caucasian or Asian?
2. Do you have a family history of osteoporosis?
3. Are you a postmenopausal woman?
4. Have you had a hysterectomy (your uterus removed)? An oophorectomy (your ovaries removed)? Both?
5. Have you been taking thyroid medication or cortisonelike drugs for asthma, arthritis, chronic skin disease, or cancer?
6. Is your diet low in dairy products and other sources of calcium?
7. ARE YOU PHYSICALLY INACTIVE?
8. Do you now, or have you ever smoked?

Please see Chapter 10 on osteoporosis.

Calcium Content of Some Foods (in milligrams)

Skim milk (1 cup)	300	Sardines in oil	350
Yogurt, nonfat (1 c)	450	Green leafy veggies*	
Yogurt, low fat (1 c)	415	Broccoli (1 c)	94
Evaporated skim milk (1 c)	265	Collards (1 c)	357
Parmesan cheese (10 oz.)	275	Taco	220
Yogurt cheese (1/2 c)	240	Almonds (1 c)	332
Monterey jack cheese, low fat (1 oz.)	225		
Swiss cheese, low fat (1 oz.)	200		
Mozzarella cheese, part-skim (1/2 c)	150	(Agricultural Handbook,	
Ricotta cheese lt. (1/2 c)	135	U.S. Dept. of Agr.)	
Cottage cheese, nonfat (1/2 cup)	60	*The darker the green, the more the calcium.	

Fiber Content of Some Foods

The recommended amount of fiber in the diet is 20 to 30 grams per day. Start slowly. There is one gram of fiber per level tablespoon (T) of bran. Bran products are available in tablets, cookies, and wafers!

All Bran cereal (2/3 cup)	18.0 grams
Fiber One cereal (1 oz.)	13.0 grams
Pinto beans (1/2 cup)	2.4 grams
Green peas (1/2 cup)	5.5 grams
Apple, with skin (1 med.)	3.0 grams
Wheaties cereal (1 oz.)	3.0 grams
Raisins (3 T)	2.0 grams
Raspberries (1/2 cup)	6.8 grams
Peanuts (1/4 cup)	3.0 grams
Shredded Wheat (2/3 cup)	3.6 grams
Prunes (3)	3.7 grams
Whole-wheat bread (2 slices)	4.0 grams
Pear (1 med.)	4.2 grams

A way to take lots of fiber and help avoid constipation is to mix 1 cup apple sauce, 1 cup miller's bran, and 1/2 cup prune juice together. Take 1 to 3 tablespoons daily. You get approximately 5 to 7 grams of fiber per tablespoon. Keep it refrigerated. Remarkably good.

References:

"Robert C. Palmer, M.D." Albuquerque *Journal,* "Trends" section, April 20, 1992.

"Focus On Fiber." Brochure from General Mills, Box 1112 Dept. 90, Minneapolis, MN 55440.

Appendix K

Basal Metabolic Rate

Your basal metabolic rate (BMR), or the minimum amount of energy needed to keep your body at its present size, is approximately your weight times 10. For example: if your weight is 140 pounds, you need 1,400 calories from food just to maintain your body <u>at rest.</u>

You must then add 30 percent more calories (1,400 + 420 = 1,820 calories) so that you will have a supply of energy great enough for your <u>normal daily activities.</u>

> EXAMPLE: Your weight times 10 = ?
>
> ? times 0.3 = ??
>
> ? + ?? = X (the calories you must have to maintain your normal daily activity level)

If you arrange <u>extra</u> activity, exercise, or chores--enough to use an extra 200 "activity calories" per day--you will benefit by losing fat and gaining muscle.

If you want to lose weight faster, then eat less than, for example, 1,820 "food calories," and exercise **too**, and you will <u>double</u> the effect!

You must be careful to lose fat at only about one pound per week, because your body will "reset" your BMR <u>lower</u> in order to defend itself against "starvation"!

Fat contains twice the calories per gram (9) than do protein (4) and carbohydrate (4). Therefore, eating less fat, gram for gram, is twice as efficient in decreasing your caloric intake. The BONUS is that you eat less of the food (fat) that is most dangerous to you.

One-half to one pound per week of weight loss is quite fast enough--after all, you are planning for a lifetime, and 26 to 52 pounds would be a <u>great</u> start the first year.

Appendix L

Some Food Items of about 250 Calories

I was astonished to discover that each one of these items contained all the calories I needed to cut out of a day's eating. Just one Snickers bar or one serving of french fries less, and you'll have accomplished today's goal! There are hundreds of other food items like these--especially snacks. Read the labels on some of your favorites and find out how easily you can drop all 200 calories at once.

Food	Calories
Big MAC	215
Small fries	220
Danish pastry	275
Snickers bar	260
Potatoes, fried (1 cup)	240
Potato chips (20)	230
Applesauce (1 cup)	230
Peanuts, salted (1½ oz.)	280
Potatoes, mashed (1 cup)	240
Cocoa, whole milk (8 oz.)	235
Oysters, fried (6)	250
Cheesecake (1 wedge)	250
Peanut butter & jelly sandwich	275
Beef, roast (3½ oz.)	260

M. Your Heart Rate, Ranges and Zones

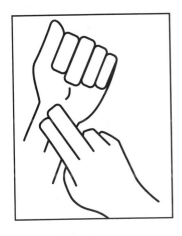

Heart Rate is measured in Beats Per Minute (BPM).

To calculate your **Maximum Heart Rate**, which is the most rapidly you should allow your heart to beat, subtract your age from220.

220 minus age = MHR (BPM)
Example: 220-40= 180 (BPM)

To find **Target Heart Rate**, which is the rate at which you can **most safely** increase your heart and lung action, follow along:

1. Glance back at chapter 16 **Thinking about Goals**: pick a "%".

2. Find your age at the left, move across chart to the "%" you have chosen: <u>GO STRAIGHT UP</u> to the top line, to find your Target Heart Rate. Work at 5-10 beats faster or slower; 20 min, 3-5 times a week.

TARGET HEART RATE

AGE	MHR	72	80	100	120	140	160
75	145		X	X	X	X	
70	150		X	X	X	X	
65	155		X	X	X	X	
60	160		X	X	X	X	
55	165		X	X	X	X	
50	170		X	X	X	X	
45	175	HEALTH	X	X	X		
40	180		X	X	X	X	
35	185		X	X	X	X	X
30	190		X	X	X	X	X
25	195		X	X	X	X	X
20	200		X	X	X	X	X
% of MHR		50%		60%	70%		80%
EFFORT=		Light		Medium	Hard		Harder

SECONDS TO COUNT:

	60	15	10	6
THR				
160	40	27	16	
150	38	25	15	
140	35	23	14	
130	33	22	13	
120	30	20	12	
110	28	18	11	
100	25	17	10	
90	23	15	9	
80	20	13	8	
73	18	12	7	

FITNESS

ATHLETE

Appendix N

Nutrition Facts: The New Label

(FDA *Medical Bulletin,* vol. 24, no. 1, May 1994)

Nutrition Facts
Serving Size   1/2 cup (114g)
Servings Per Container   4

← Standard, sensible "human" size servings.

Amount Per Serving
Calories 260   Calories from Fat 120

← Generally look for a big difference between the numbers. "Calories from Fat", multiplied by three, should be less than "Calories. If a serving contains more than 5 grams of fat, avoid it. Total fat for the day 50-65 gm.

	% Daily Value
Total Fat 13 gms	20%
Saturated Fat 5 gm	25%
Cholesterol 30 mg	10%
Sodium 660 mg	28%
Total Carbohydrate 31 gm	11%
Dietary Fiber 0g	0%
Sugars 5g	
Protein 5g	

Viatmin A	4%	Vitamin C	2%
Calcium	15%	Iron	4%

← These four are required. Some will offer more items.

*Percent Daily Values are based on a 2,000-calorie diet. your daily values may be higher or lower depending on your calorie needs:

← 2,000 Cals. About 150 pounds.

	Calories	2,000	2,500
Total Fat	Less than	65g	80g
Sat Fat	Less than	20g	25g
Cholesterol	Less than	300mg	300mg
Sodium	Less than	2,400mg	2,400mg
Total Carbohydrate		25g	30g

← On all labels. If you wish to figure YOUR daily calorie needs see Appendix K. ((BMR).

Calories per gram:
   Fat 9 • Carbohydrate 4 • Protein 4

← Basic Reference. On most labels.

Appendix O

Your Doctor Partner

Please invite your doctor to read this message from the Greater Albuquerque Medical Association and the New Mexico Governor's Council on Health, Physical Fitness, and Sports.

Despite the public's recognized value of physical activity, only 22% of Americans are active at the levels recommended for good health. Consequently, America's physical inactivity has a significant impact on the health of the nation and the staggering cost of health care. Specifically, over 250,000 deaths each years can be attributed to lack of physical activity.

To combat the problem, the American College of Sports Medicine (ACSM), the U.S. Centers for Disease Control and Prevention, along with the President's Council on Physical Fitness and Sports, have issued new recommendations for the amount of exercise needed for good health: "Every American adult should accumulate 30 minutes or more of moderate intensity physical activity over the course of most days of the week."

You are in a powerful position to play an integral role in helping implement these new recommendations by counseling your patients on the new guidelines. Research by the National Center for Health Statistics shows that even modestly effective physician counseling would have a substantial public health impact on improving activity levels. To assist your effort, the Greater Albuquerque Medical Association in conjunction with the New Mexico Governor's Council for Health, Physical Fitness, and Sports and local representatives of the American College of Sports Medicine Healthy People 2000 volunteer network have worked together to produce a physical activity recommendation form for patient activity.

The recommendation that this person brings to you has been carefully reviewed to meet standards of good patient education as well as the recommendations from the American College of Sports Medicine. If you or one of your personnel in your office can take a few minutes to go over this form and work through it together with your patient, effective counseling can be accomplished. When your knowledge of your patient is added into the recommendations and guidelines, it will have a great impact upon your patient to become more active in daily life. We believe this is much more effective than just simply handing out a brochure and leaving them on their own to figure it out.

Please copy this form as much as you wish and use it freely.

If you have any questions or want to talk to any of us about this new recommendation form, please feel free to call GAMA at 505-821-4583 or Dr. George Dixon at 505-344-8755 (home and FAX).

Sincerely,

George L. Dixon, M.D.,
Governor's Council for
Health Physical Fitness &
Sports
Chris McGrew, M.D.,
Chair,GAMA Sports
Medicine Committee
& ACSM Healthy
People 2000
State Representative
Peg Allen,
District Health Office
Virginia Crenshaw,
GCHPF & S
Luis Curet, M.D., UNM
Dept of OB/GYN

Eugene Dix, GCHPF & S
Christian Meuli, M.D.,
NM Chapter, American
Academy of Family Practice
Mike Nelson, M.D.,
GAMA Sports
Medicine Committee
Jo Ann Ortiz,
NM Department of Health
Albert Rizzoli, M.D.,
NM Chapter, American
Society of Internal Medicine
Joanne Sprenger,
NMAHPERD

PHYSICAL ACTIVITY RECOMMENDATIONS
FOR A HEALTHIER YOU!

BENEFITS OF PHYSICAL ACTIVITY FOR YOU:

✓ Increase your energy ✓ Improve your mood ✓ Maintain or lose weight✓ Improve sleep✓ Decrease daily aches and pains✓ Reduce stress ✓ Prevent, control, or reverse diabetes ✓ Protect yourself against heart disease and some kinds of cancer.

Name two main benefits you hope to get from being physically active:

PHYSICAL ACTIVITY MUST BE REGULAR
- ✓ For most days of the week, aim to accumulate 30 minutes or more of light, moderate, or vigorous activities over the day.
- ✓ Plan to do physical activities of your choice at least 3 - 5 days each week, and let these activities become your habits.
- ✓ Note your activities on your calendar to keep a record.

ACTIVITIES   Circle the activities you will do.

Light	Moderate	Vigorous
Gardening	Brisk walking	Swimming laps
Play catch with children	Mall walking	Fast cycling
Park farther away than usual	Walking upstairs	Jogging/running
Walk to work	Ice/roller skating	Aerobic dance
Piñon/fruit picking	Dancing	Basketball
	Juggling	Singles tennis
	Chopping wood	Racquet sports
		Soccer
	River fishing	Martial arts
	Water exercise	
	Recreational swimming	
	Hiking	
	Slow cycling	
	Doubles tennis	

. . . and any other physical activities you enjoy

PLANNING helps:
Where will you do your activities?

Who will help you and how?

What are the best times of the day?

Challenges and common problems and solutions in getting started:
How will I fit this into my day?
    Do it with family members. Do some of your 30 minutes on your way to work, on the job, or around the house.

I've never been good at sports.
   Many of these activities are NOT sports. Select activities you like!
I'm usually too tired to exercise.
   Regular activity improves your energy level. Try it and see.
Exercise is boring.
   Do it with somebody. Listen to music. Enjoy the beautiful New Mexico vistas.
I get sore when I exercise.
   Mild muscle soreness that lasts 2 - 3 days is common when getting started. Build up gradually and stretch before and after physical activity.
It's too expensive.
   The only equipment needed is a good pair of sturdy, comfortable shoes, which may already be in your closet.

Are you ready to go?

Yes	No	
O	O	Has a doctor ever said that you have a heart condition and recommended medically supervised activity?
O	O	Do you have chest pain brought on by physical activity?
O	O	Have you developed chest pain in the past month?
O	O	Do you tend to lose consciousness or fall over as a result of dizziness?
O	O	Do you have a bone or joint problem that could be aggravated by the proposed physical activity?
O	O	Has a doctor ever recommended medication for your high blood pressure or heart condition?
O	O	Are you aware through your own experience, or a doctor's advice, of any other physical reasons against your exercising without medical supervision?

   If you answered yes to any of these questions, discuss this with your physician before starting or increasing physical activity.

**The New Mexico Governor's Council on Health,
Physical Fitness, and Sports
and the
Greater Albuquerque Medical Association**
1994
Inspiration from the American College of Sports Medicine
"Exercise Lite" Program and the
Physician Assessment & Counseling for
Exercise Program (P.A.C.E.),
University of California, San Diego.

SOURCES

Introduction

"National Fitness Study 1989." National Sporting Goods Association.

"Healthy People 2000: Physical Activity Objectives." U.S. Department of Health and Human Services.

Live Longer Cookbook. Reader's Digest Association, Pleasantville, NY. 1992.

Chapter 1

Healthy People 2000. U.S. Department of Health and Human Services.

"The Benefits of Regular Exercise." IRSA. The Association of Quality Clubs, Boston, MA 02210. 1991.

Biomarkers: The Ten Keys for Prolonging Vitality. William J. Evans, Ph.D. Fireside Books, New York.

"Are You Getting Enough Sleep?" University of Texas *Lifetime Health Letter,* vol. 5, no. 8, August 1993.

"The Beauty of Strength." Mary Lisa Gavenas. *Weight Watcher's Magazine,* March 1993.

"Exercise for Good Sex." *Arch. of Sexual Behavior,* vol. 19, no. 3, 1990. Quoted in *Edell Health Letter,* February 1991.

"Getting Quality Sleep." Daniel Blackwood, M.A. In *Employee Assistance Program,* Fall 1992.

"Fit Facts: The Healthy Side Effects of Exercise and Activity." The National Exercise For Life Institute, Excelsior, MN 55331-9967. 1993.

Home Fitness Journal, vol. 2, no. 2. CVT Productions, Inc., Eugene, OR 97401.

Running and FitNews, vol. 11, no. 3, March 1993. American Running and Fitness Association, Bethesda, MD 20814.

University of Texas *Lifetime Health Letter,* January 1992. Palm Coast, FL 32142-0342.

Chapter 2

"Strength Conditioning." Frances Munnings. *The Physician and Sports Medicine.,* vol. 21, no. 4, April 1993.

The Performance Edge. Robert K. Cooper. Houghton Mifflin, Boston. Quoted in *Bottom Line Personal,* February 1992.

Personal note. Jennifer D. Hamilton, R.P.T.

Chapter 3

Fitness Without Exercise. Bryant Stamford, Ph.D., and Porter Shiner. Warner Books, New York. 1990.

The Exercise Exchange Program. Dr. James M. Rippe, with Patricia Amend. Simon and Schuster, New York. 1992.

Chapter 4

The Exercise Exchange Program. Dr. James M. Rippe, with Patricia Amend. Simon and Schuster, New York. 1992.

"The 10 Minute Workout." Nancy Gagliardi. *Weight Watcher's Women's Health and Fitness News,* October 1990.

"Walk Your Way to Feeling Better" and "Getting Stronger by Using Weights." Patient Handouts. *The Physician and Sportsmedicine,* vol. 21, no. 2, February 1993.

"Boosting Abdominal Strength without Back Pain." Patient Handout. *The Physician and Sportsmedicine,* vol. 21, no. 4, April 1993.

"Exercises for the Abdominal Muscles." Posted on bulletin board at the O'Hare Health and Racquet Club at the Westin O'Hare Hotel. From Parkside Sport and Fitness Center, a division of Lutheran General Health Care System, Park Ridge, IL.

"Balance Training Can Help Keep Elderly on Feet." Ira Dreyfuss. Associated Press. Albuquerque *Journal,* March 2, 1992.

"Stretching." Jennifer Hamilton, R.P.T. *Home Fitness Journal,* vol. 2, no. 1, 1992. Published by CVT Productions, Inc., Eugene, OR 97401.

"Stretching." Bill Laitner. Knight-Ridder Newspapers. Albuquerque *Journal,* 1992.

Better Bodies after 35. Irving Beychok, M.D. Published by Mills and Sanderson, Bedford, MA 01730. Quoted in *Bottom Line Personal.*

"Your Patient and Fitness." Fitness Tip. Strong and Flexible. Patient Handout. *The Physician and Sports Medicine.* Vol. 5, no. 4, July/August 1991.

"Proper Stretching Order." Letter by Douglas Lentz, CSCS, Chamberberg, PA. In *Running and Fitness News,* vol. 11, no. 7.

"Basic Training: Guide to Muscle Making." Supplement to *Men's Fitness,* August 1993.

"Exercise for Health." John R. Sallade, P.T. American Physical Therapy Association. *Clinical Management in Physical Therapy,* vol. 6, no. 1, January/Febuary 1986.

"Slideboards." A presentation at American College of Sports Medicine, Seattle, WA, 1993, by H. N. Williford, Ed.D., and R. M. Otto,

Ph.D. Reported in *Running and FitNews,* vol. 11, no. 10, October 1993.

Fitness Without Exercise. Bryant Stamford, Ph.D., and Porter Shiner. Warner Books, New York. 1990.

Chapter 5

Home Fitness Journal, vol. 2, no. 2, 1992.

"Home Exercise Equipment: Comparing Aerobic-Exercise Equipment." University of California at Berkeley *Wellness Letter,* December 1992.

"Walk Your Way to Fitness." Press Release. American Running and Fitness Association, Bethesda, MD 20814.

"The Other Kind of Exercise." Special Report. Tufts University *Diet and Nutrition Letter,* vol. 11, no. 5, July 1993.

"Get Fit at Any Age." Senior fitness note, *European Journal of Applied Physiology,* vol. 65, pp. 203 - 208. Quoted in *Running and FitNews,* vol. 11, no. 7, July 1993.

"Water Workouts." *Home Fitness Journal,* vol. 3, no. 1, 1993. CVT Productions, Eugene, OR 97401.

"Fitness Update." "Afterburn." "Treading Water." *Consumer Reports on Health,* vol. 5, no. 10, October 1993.

Chapter 6

"Exercises You Can Take to Work." Mary P. Schatz. Adapted from her book, *Back Care Basics.* Rodmell Press, Berkeley, CA. Patient handout in *The Physician and Sportsmedicine,* vol. 20, no. 1, January 1992.

"Fitness You Can Pack: Running Away From Home." Peter Jaret. *Health,* April 1992.

Chapter 7

"The New Yoga." Daryl Eller. *American Health,* July/August 1993.

"Yoga Tones Up Mind and Body." Ralph LaForge, M.Sc. *Executive Health's Good Health Report,* vol. 29, no. 11, August 1993.

"The Soft Side of Exercise." Daryl Eller. *Walking Magazine,* November/December 1992.

"Quiet Strength: T'ai Chi." Kathryn Keller. *Men's Health,* March/April 1993.

Chapter 8

"Eating More Vegetables: Update." *Weight Watchers Magazine,* March 1993.

"The Food Guide Pyramid." U.S. Department of Agriculture. U.S. Department of Health and Human Services.

Understanding Weight Loss. The National Exercise for Life Institute, Excelsior, MN 55331-9967.

Willpower To Go. Laura Terroux. Applewood Press. Quoted in *Weight Watcher's Magazine,* March 1993.

"Weight Management and Body Image." University of Texas *Lifetime Health Letter,* vol. 5, no. 13, November 1993.

The New Fit or Fat. Covert Bailey. Houghton Mifflin Company, Boston. 1991.

Eat More, Weigh Less. Dean Ornish, M.D. Harper Collins, New York. 1993.

"Weight Loss Workouts: The Stationary Cycling Workout Guide and Log." Cycle Vision Tours, Inc., Eugene, OR 97401.

Fit or Fat Target Recipes. Covert Bailey and Lea Bishop. Houghton Mifflin, Boston. 1985.

"Fat Burning Workouts." Ralph LaForge, M.Sc. *Executive Health's Good Health Report,* February 1993.

"Eating for Energy." Debra Waterhouse, M.P.H., R.D. *Weight Watchers Magazine,* March 1993.

"How Much Fat Do You Have?" Dr. John McMahon. Quoted in University of Texas *Lifetime Health Letter.* 1992.

"Glossing the Fat." Elizabeth N. Hiser, M.S., R.D. *Eating Well Magazine,* September/October 1991.

"Fiber Primer." In "Walking Shorts." *Walking Magazine,* March/April 1992.

Nutritive Value of Foods. Home and Garden Bulletin no. 72. U.S. Department of Agriculture, Human Nutrition Information Services, Washington, DC. 1986.

"Burning More Fat during Exercise." Presentations by Peggy Arnos, M.S., et. al., and by F. A. Kulling, M.S., at the annual meeting of the American College of Sports Medicine, Seattle, WA, June 2 - 5, 1993. Reported in *Running and FitNews,* vol. 11, no. 11, November 1993. American Running and Fitness Association, Bethesda, MD 20814.

"Weight-Loss Guidelines." Jeffery Fisher, M.D. Quoted in *Bottom Line Personal,* vol. 14, no. 21, November 15, 1993.

"Exercise, Obesity, and Weight Control." Guest author, Jack H. Wilmore. *Physical Activity and Fitness Research Digest,* series 1, no. 6, May 1994. President's Council on Physical Fitness and Sports.

Chapter 9

"How Much Should I Exercise?" Bryant Stamford, PhD. *The Physician and Sportsmedicine,* vol. 17, no. 7, July 1989.

"Contraindicated Exercises." Ruth Sova, M.S. *The AKWA Letter,* vol. 7, no. 2, August 1993. Aquatic Exercise Association.

"Avoiding Overuse Injury." Ralph LaForge, M.Sc. *Executive Health's Good Health Report,* April 1993.

MAYO Clinical Update, pp. 5 - 6, 1993.

"Back Savers." From *The Back Almanac.* Lanier Publishing, Oakland, CA 94620. Quoted in *Bottom Line Personal,* August 30, 1993.

"Fighting Back Pain." Julia Califano. *Weight Watcher's Magazine,* December, 1992.

Healing Back Pain. John Sarno, M.D. Warner Books, New York.

"Taking the Pain Out of Work." Mary Anne Dunkin. *Arthritis Today,* January/February 1993. The Arthritis Foundation, Inc.

"Repetitive Motion--How Much Is Too Much?" Langford Physical Therapy, Albuquerque, NM 87108. December 1991.

"Carpal Tunnel Syndrome: Wrist Problems Arise at Home or Work." University of Texas *Lifetime Health Letter,* vol. 6, no. 7, July 1994.

"Hazards of the High-Tech Workplace." Laura B. Kaufman. *Weight Watcher's Women's Health and Fitness News,* October 1990.

"Lift It Safe!" Brochure. American Academy of Orthopaedic Surgeons, 6300 N. River Rd., Rosemont, IL 60018.

"Heart Rate and Exertion." Ralph LaForge, M.Sc. *Executive Health's Good Health Report,* vol. 29, no. 12, September 1993.

"Fitness File: Pulse Finding." *Men's Confidential,* vol. 9, no. 10, October 1993.

Chapter 10

"Osteoarthritis." *Home Fitness Journal,* vol. 3, no. 1, 1993. CVT Productions, Inc., Eugene, OR 97401.

"Exercise Is the Best Medicine." Ralph LaForge, M.Sc. *Executive Health's Good Health Report,* March 1992.

"Exercising Safely (with Rheumatoid Arthritis)." *Consumer Reports on Health,* vol. 5, no. 9, September 1993.

"Diabetes and Exercise." James R. Gavin III, M.D. *American Journal of Nursing,* February 1988.

"Risk of Diabetes." The John's Hopkins Medical Letter, *Health after 50.* Quoted in *Bottom Line Personal,* April 30, 1993.

"Exercise and Its Benefits." In "People with Diabetes: Getting Started." Booklet. Becton Dickinson and Company. 1985.

"Fat and Diabetes." In "Nutrition Update." *Consumer Reports on Health,* August 1993.

"Exercise and Diabetes." *Home Fitness Journal,* vol. 2, no. 3, 1992. CVT Productions, Inc., Eugene, OR 97401.

"Your Blood Pressure." Larry Katzenstein. *American Health,* June 1992.

"New Guidelines for Hypertension." Amber Stenger. *The Physician and Sportsmedicine,* vol. 21, no. 2, February 1993.

Guidelines for Exercise Testing and Prescription. American College of Sports Medicine. Fourth Edition. Lea and Febiger, Philadelphia and London. 1991.

"Fight High Blood Pressure." *Health Break,* September 1993. New Heart, Albuquerque, NM 87108.

"A Lifelong Program to Build Strong Bones." University of California at Berkeley *Wellness Letter,* vol. 9, no. 10, July 1993.

"Bone Up on Your Diet." Susan M. Kleiner, Ph.D, R.D. *The Physician and Sportsmedicine,* vol. 21, no. 5, May 1993.

The Mars One Crew Manual. Kerry Mark Joels. Ballentine Books, New York. 1985.

"Live It Safe." Brochure from the American Academy of Orthopaedic Surgeons, 6300 N. River Rd., Rosemont, IL 60018. 1993.

"Guide to a Healthy Pregnancy." *Health+Plus News,* 1993. 7500 Jefferson NE, Albuquerque, NM 87109.

"Exercising for Two." In "Fitness Update." *Consumer Reports on Health,* August 1993.

"Exercise during Pregnancy and the Postpartum Period." ACOG *Technical Bulletin,* no. 189, February 1994.

"Exercising for Two. What's Safe?" Jaqueline White. *The Physician and Sportsmedicine,* vol. 20, no. 5, May 1992.

"Babies Prefer Pre-Exercise Breast Milk." *Pediatrics,* vol. 89, no. 6, pp. 1245 - 47. Reported in *Running and FitNews,* vol. 11, no. 3, March 1993. American Running and Fitness Association.

"Postpartum Pounds No Cause for the Blues." National Center for Health Statistics. Reported in Tufts University *Diet and Nutrition Letter,* vol. 11, no. 8, October 1993.

"Staying Active in Cold Weather." Brochure. American Running and Fitness Association, Bethesda, MD.

"No-Excuse Holiday Exercises." Ralph LaForge, M.Sc. *Executive Health's Good Health Report,* vol. 29, no. 3, December 1992.

"Enjoying Winter Exercise." Press Release. American Running and Fitness Association, Bethesda, MD.

"Extra Vitamin D in Winter?" Robban Sica-Cohen, M.D. Quoted in *Bottom Line Personal,* January 30, 1993.

"Chill vs. Will." Gary Legwold. *Bicycle Guide Magzine,* February 1992.

"How to Freeze Your Buns Off." Annette Spence. *Walking Magazine,* January/February 1993.

"Hot Weather, Exercise, and You." Brochure. American Running and Fitness Association, Bethesda, MD.

Chapter 11

"Home Gym on a Shoestring." The University of Texas *Lifetime Health Letter,* 1992.

"The Best Workout? Free Weights vs. Machines." The University of California at Berkeley *Wellness Letter,* March 1993.

"Skipping Exercise." *Men's Health,* June 1992.

The Indoor Bicycling Fitness Program. Jane S. Peters. McGraw-Hill Book Company, New York. 1985.

"Exercise, Obesity, and Weight Control." Guest author Jack H. Wilmore. *Physical Activity and Fitness Research Digest,* series 1, no. 6, May 1994. President's Council on Physical Fitness and Sports.

Chapter 12

Fitness and Fallacies. Rick DeLorme, M.A., M.S., and Fred Stransky, Ph.D. Kendall/Hunt Publishing Company, Dubuque, IA 52004-0539.

"Exercise Best Investment." J. Phillip Dickinson. *The Retirement Letter,* February 1993.

"Home Exercise Equipment: Comparisons of Machines." University of California at Berkeley *Wellness Letter,* December 1992.

Banish Your Potbelly. Editors of *Men's Health.* Rodale Press, Inc., Emmaus, PA 18098.

"Fighting Winter's Flabby Muscles." *Longevity,* February 1993.

"The Best Workout? Free Weights vs. Machines." University of California at Berkeley *Wellness Letter,* March 1993.

The Weight Training Workbook. Jim Bennett. JBBA Publishing, Inc., Menasha, WI. l991. Distributor: 800-345-0096.

Chapter 13

"A Walker's Guide to Fitness Videos." Susanna Levin. *Walking Magazine,* January/February 1993.

"Sixth Annual Fitness Video Review." *Shape,* January 1993.

"The New Men's Gym." David Rosenbaum. *Longevity,* September 1993

"Influence of Video Assisted Cycling on Self Selected Exercise Intensity." Robert A. Robergs, Ph.D., and Mellissa Knight, M.S. Research Report. Center for Exercise and Applied Human Physiology, University of New Mexico, Albuquerque, NM 87113.

"The Best Exercise Videos." Peg Jordan, R.N. *Bottom Line Personal,* August 15, 1993.

"Third Annual Exercise Video Awards." *Self,* March 1993.

"The Exercise Standards and Malpractice Reporter." January 1992. Quoted in *Executive Health's Good Health Report,* September 1992.

Chapter 14

"Don't Be an Exercise Dropout." Sue Browder. *Reader's Digest,* August 1991.

"Identifying the Salient Outcomes of Exercise: Application of Marketing Principles to Preventive Health Behavior." Elizabeth C. Schmelling, R.N., Ph.D. *Public Health Nursing,* vol. 2, no. 2, June 1985.

"Motivation Hints". Home Fitness Journal, vol. 1, nos. 1 - 2, l991. CVT Productions, Inc.

"Put Your Money Where Your Mouth Is." "Men's Health, December 1991.

"Exercise for a Lifetime!" Brochure. Produced for Geico Insurance Company by American Running and Fitness Association, Bethesda, MD.

"Tips to Avoid Exercise Staleness." Ralph LaForge, M.Sc. *Executive Health's Good Health Report,* vol. 29, no. 9, June 1993.

Chapter 15

"Massage: Benefits and Pleasures." University of California at Berkeley *Wellness Letter,* October 1992.

"Blissful Relaxation: Underwater Massage." Nancy Wartik. *Self,* March 1993.

"Relaxation: An Important Part of Fitness." Donya Currie. Knight-Ridder Newspapers. Abuquerque *Journal,* January 4, 1993.

"Make Yourself Happier." Paul Ekman, Ph.D., In *Pyschological Science,* 40 West 20th St., New York, NY 10011. Reported in *Bottom Line Personal,* March 1, 1994.

"Help Yourself: Massage, Self Administered and Sports Massage." *Running and FitNews,* vol. 11, no. 5, 1993. American Running and Fitness Association.

"Stress: What You Can Do About It." Albuquerque *Journal,* September 20, 1993.

INDEX